The Facts On File
Dictionary of Fitness

The Facts On File Dictionary of Fitness

By Ardy Friedberg

Facts On File Publications
New York, New York • Bicester, England

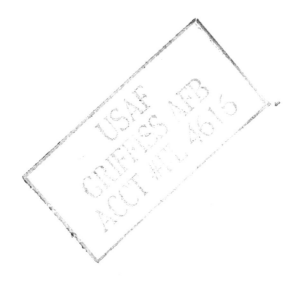

The Facts On File Dictionary of Fitness

Library of Congress Cataloging in Publication Data

Friedberg, Ardy.
    The Facts on File dictionary of fitness.
    1. Physical fitness—Dictionaries.   I. Title.
GV481.F73   1984   613.7'03   83-1592
ISBN 0-87196-809-6

Printed in the United States of America

10 9 8 7 6 5 4 3 2 1

For my Dad

Introduction

The fitness movement that began in this country in the early 1970s has been with us for more than a decade now. As societal changes go it has not been as dramatic as some of the events of the same period; nevertheless, it has had a profound impact on the lifestyles of millions of people, and the message of health and fitness that it developed is now part of the fabric of our society.

Historically, the genesis of the movement can be traced to the 1972 Olympics, when Frank Shorter, an unknown American runner, won the gold medal in the marathon. His surprising victory seemed to strike the right chord at the right time, and almost immediately joggers by the thousands appeared on the streets and byways as if in search of some distant Olympic medal. For the most part these runners were ordinary people, not athletes, who were inspired by the force of Shorter's example and quickly became convinced there was something inherently rewarding and important about staying fit.

The national mania for fitness gathered momentum in the mid-1970s when Dr. Kenneth Cooper discovered "aerobics." Then Jim Fixx created a quantum leap in public awareness with *The Complete Book of Running*, a layman's approach to long-distance running that sprinted to the top of the best-seller list.

By the end of the decade, medical researchers confirmed what active exercisers had felt and hoped was the case: that exercise had a positive effect on health, well-being, mental acuity, and that just possibly, it also increases longevity. This laboratory proof of the efficacy of exercise formed the permanent foundation that has supported the revolution, and today pollsters estimate that 75 million Americans exercise on a regular basis.

This deep national interest in health, diet, and physical fitness has created its own growth industries in clothing, shoes, equipment of all kinds, and a proliferation of information on the subject in the form of books, special-interest magazines, and audio and video tapes. At the same time, the new world of fitness also created the elements of a new language, a jargon that was formed by a combination of words in new contexts (i.e., personal best, overload and cooldown) and the popularizing of words and phrases that have been the exclusive province of athletes, coaches, doctors, and nutritionists (i.e., plantar fasciitis, dynamometer, and carbohydrate loading).

This book defines these fitness-related terms. The words and phrases in this volume were selected from thousands in current usage because they comprise the essential elements of an adequate fitness vocabulary. They are arranged alphabetically and cross-referenced for convenience. In many cases additional information is provided that goes beyond a standard dictionary definition.

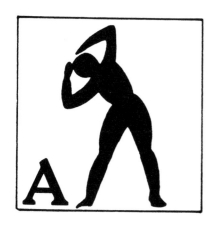

abdomen

The part of the body in mammals that lies between the thorax and the pelvis and encloses the viscera, or internal organs of the body (commonly called the intestines); the belly.

abdominal board

A special bench designed to isolate the abdominal muscles in such exercises as the sit-up; usually can be angled from 0 to 45°.

abdominal cramps

See *dysmenorrhea.*

abdominal muscles

The three muscles attached to the front and sides of the rib cage and the pelvis. Their purpose is to stabilize the pelvis and chest so that other muscles can move the arms and legs or parts of the trunk in desired movements. They also retract the abdomen to hold the viscera in place and are associated with the action of the diaphragm in breathing. The three muscles involved are the rectus abdominis in the center of the stomach area, the external oblique on the lower front of the rib cage, and the internal oblique that sits next to it.

abdominals

The muscles of the abdominal area, including the rectus abdominis, and the external oblique and internal oblique muscles that attach to the ribs (see *abdominal muscles*).

abdominous

Potbellied.

abduct

The movement of a part of the body away from the midline of the body; the arm, in abduction, is raised; abduct is the opposite of adduct (see *adduct*).

able-bodied

Being physically strong and healthy.

abrasion

Injury to the first layer of the skin.

abs

The slang term used by bodybuilders and other exercisers for the abdominals or stomach muscles; also "abbies," as in "washboard abbies."

acceleration sprints

The increase in speed from jogging to short bursts of sprinting, during which distances may range from 50 to 400 yards or more; a variation of "wind sprints," which are all-out, short-duration sprints of 40 to 60 yards.

acclimatization

The physiological adjustments brought about through continued exposure to a different climate or altitude, as when athletes train at high altitudes for sports events that will take place at those altitudes.

acetylcholine

A chemical substance (ACh) involved in several important physiological functions, including transmission of an impulse from one nerve fiber to another across a synapse; the motor nerve is an example of a nerve that communicates with other nerves and with the skeletal muscles by means of ACh; choline is formed when ACh breaks down.

Achilles tendon

The large tendon running from the heel bone to the calf muscle of the leg, which is vital to easy movement. Injury to the tendon can immobilize an athlete or an exerciser for an indefinite time.

ACTH

Called the "alarm messenger" hormone, it causes the adrenal glands to release epinephrine, norepinephrine, and cortisones; this release results in a speed-up of heart rate and respiration, release of sugar from the liver and release of fatty acids into the blood, and it causes the muscles to tense.

actin

A protein found in the muscles that, with myosin, activates muscular contraction.

active

In action; moving; leading a non-sedentary life in which a person participates in a variety of pursuits.

actomyosin

A combination of actin and myosin that, with other substances, constitutes muscle fiber and is responsible for muscular contraction and expansion.

acupuncture

An Oriental method of treatment for muscular tension and a variety of other ailments from flu to insomnia; involves the insertion of needles into the skin at precisely predetermined points; in some cases the needles are turned and twisted to achieve the desired result; generally little or no pain is involved.

adduct

To pull or draw a part of the body toward the midline of the body; the raised arm, when lowered is adducted. This is the opposite of abduct (see *abduct*).

adenosine diphosphate (ADP)

A complex chemical compound which, when combined with inorganic phosphate, forms ATP; part of the phosphagen system and one of the building blocks for ATP synthesis (see *adenosine triphosphate*).

adenosine triphosphate (ATP)
A complex chemical compound that is formed with the energy released from food and stored in all cells, particularly muscle cells; the immediately usable form of chemical energy for muscular activity; the breakdown of this compound enables the cells to perform work (see *adenosine diphosphate*).

adipocyte
A cell that stores fat.

adipose tissue
Fatty tissue; approximately 15% of body tissue is adipose in men and approximately 25% in women.

adiposis
Excessive body fat; liposis.

ADP
See *adenosine diphosphate (ADP)*.

aerobic dancing
Exercise consisting of a mixture of rhythmic running, hopping, skipping, jumping, sliding, stretching, and swinging, as well as a number of dance steps; the creation of this form of exercise is credited to Jackie Sorenson, an exercise specialist with a background in dance.

aerobic metabolism
A series of chemical reactions taking place in the body and requiring oxygen.

aerobic power
The ability to take in and use oxygen during physical work; maximal aerobic power (VO_2max), while highly individualized, is the greatest oxygen uptake a person can achieve; VO_2max stands for the volume (V) in liters of oxygen (O_2) used during maximal exercise. (See *VO_2max*).

aerobic training
The type of exercise that forces the pulse rate to a level sufficient to bring about a training effect (see *training effect*); if practiced for periods of 30 minutes or more three times per

week, such training improves the cardiovascular system, strengthens the heart, and improves the body's ability to deliver blood and oxygen to the muscles; activities suitable for aerobic training include rapid walking, running, swimming, bicycling, rowing, and cross-country skiing.

agility

Speed in changing body positions or direction.

Alexander Principle

One of the best known of the theories that pinpoints the spine as the center of most physical complaints. It was named for Frederick Matthias Alexander, who studied the efficient functioning of the body. The Alexander method utilizes massage as treatment.

alible

Having nutrients; nourishing.

alternate grip

A combination of the overhand and underhand methods of holding a barbell or dumbbell: one hand is palm out and the other is palm in.

amenorrhea

Menstrual irregularity, sometimes caused by regular, vigorous exercise. It is not considered dangerous.

American Alliance for Health, Physical Education, and Recreation (AAHPER)

The organization that designed the Youth Fitness Test for children 10 through 17 years of age; tests include pull-ups, bent-knee sit-ups, 40-yard shuttle run, standing broad jump, 50-yard dash, and 600-yard run-walk.

amino acids

Twenty organic, nitrogen-containing compounds that form the building blocks of protein. Capable of acting as an acid or a base, they are obtained from the diet or synthesized by living cells. There are two varieties: nonessential (manufactured by the body) and essential (obtained from food); the latter are found in most foods that contain protein (i.e., meat, fish, poultry, and eggs).

amphetamines

A variety of synthetic drugs closely related to epinephrine (adrenaline), a morphine-like substance manufactured by the body; they stimulate the central nervous system, speed up the metabolism, and reduce appetite; sometimes used by athletes for stimulation before competition and by dieters for appetite suppression.

anabolic

Tissue-building; conducive to the constructive process of metabolism; the other process of metabolism is called catabolic, meaning breaking down. Synthetic anabolic products such as anabolic steroids are used by athletes to speed and increase the construction process of the metabolism and to build muscle quickly (see *steroids*).

anaerobic

In the absence of oxygen; commonly refers to energy expenditure of short duration occurring during activities such as weight lifting or sprinting.

anaerobic glycolysis

The incomplete chemical breakdown of carbohydrate; the anaerobic reactions in this breakdown release energy for the manufacture of ATP as they produce lactic acid. Anaerobic glycolysis is also known as the lactic acid system (see *lactic acid system*).

anaerobic metabolism

A series of chemical reactions in the body that take place without the presence of oxygen.

angina pectoris

Attacks of severe chest pain resulting from an insufficient supply of blood to the heart; spasmodic attacks can be indicative of heart disease.

ankle weights

Weights, usually in the form of a cuff that is fitted around the

ankle; the additional weight is supposed to aid in training for
athletic events.

anorexia
Loss of appetite; usually the result of strict dieting and the fear
of being obese; can lead to weakness and even death; often
results in depression and anxiety.

antagonist
A muscle that opposes another muscle; the muscle that relaxes
in any movement; e.g., in flexing the elbow, the biceps muscles
contracts (prime mover) and the triceps muscle (antagonist)
relaxes (see *prime mover*).

anthropometry
The study of human body measurement; used for anthro-
pological classification and for comparison of body types;
useful in determining athletic specialization (see *somatotype*).

appestat
An area of the brain located in the hypothalamus that is
thought to control the amount of fuel coming into the body in
the form of food.

arch supports
Inserts in shoes that provide support and stabilization (see
orthotics).

arrhythmia
An uncomfortably rapid and wildly fluctuating heartbeat that
comes on in a sudden rush during or immediately following
exercise. It can occur when the exerciser stops suddenly and
usually subsides after a period of rest. Cool-down exercises
help guard against arrhythmia (see *heart block*).

arthritis
Inflammation of a joint or joints; often accompanied by fluid
accumulation and pain in the affected area; usually occurs as
part of the aging process and can be mild or severe. Athletes
sometimes develop arthritis because of the overuse of certain
joints such as the baseball pitcher's shoulder. Severe arthritis

can be immobilizing and disfiguring; exercise is helpful in many cases because it stimulates circulation.

asana
The postures or poses of yoga (see *Hatha yoga*).

Astrand, Dr. Per Olaf
Swedish work and exercise physiologist; pioneered studies in exercise physiology.

ataxia
Loss or lack of muscular coordination.

athlete
A participant in sports; a person possessing the natural pre-requisites—strength, flexibility, endurance, and special skills—for sports competition; anyone who participates in sports or fitness activities.

athlete's foot
A contagious skin infection caused by parasitic fungi (ring-worm) usually affecting the feet (and sometimes the hands) and causing itching, blisters, cracking, dryness, and scaling; usually begins in the spaces between the third and fourth toes and sometimes spreads to the soles of the feet; so named because many cases are contracted while in an athletic environment such as a locker room, shower room, or gym; a variety of creams, sprays, and ointments are available for treatment.

athletic supporter
An elastic support for the male genitals worn especially during athletic or other strenuous activity; also called a jockstrap; boxers, baseball catchers, and hockey goalies often insert a rigid metallic cup for additional protection.

Atlas, Charles
Born Angelo Siciliano, Charles Atlas is often referred to as the father of physical fitness in America. A bodybuilder and physical culturalist, he developed Dynamic Tension, an isometric-like exercise routine that has been sold through the mail since

1930. His most famous advertising phrase: "I was a 97-pound weakling."

ATP

See *adenosine triphosphate (ATP)*.

ATP-PC System

An anaerobic energy system in which adenosine triphosphate (ATP) is manufactured when phosphocreatine (PC) is broken down; this system represents the most rapidly available source of ATP for use by the muscles; activities performed at maximum intensity in a period of 10 seconds or less derive energy from the ATP system.

atrophy

The wasting away, because of inactivity, of tissues, organs, or the entire body; usually refers to the loss of strength and tone in unused muscles.

Australian crawl

A swimming stroke, a variation of the crawl executed with an eight-beat flutter kick to each stroke; also called the crawl.

autonomic nervous system

The involuntary body system that aids in controlling movement, secretion by the visceral organs, urinary output, body temperature, heart rate, blood flow, and blood pressure; termed involuntary because it functions without a person's conscious direction, e.g., it is not necessary to think about heart rate for the heart to beat (see *sympathetic nervous system*).

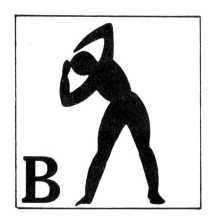

backache

See *back pain*.

back hyperextension

An exercise in which the exerciser lies face down on a bench, table, or a back-extension machine with the trunk of the body (from the waist up) extending past the end of the bench, hands clasped behind the head. The trunk is then lowered as far as possible toward the floor and raised again to the starting position, strengthening the muscles of the lower back and abdomen.

back pain

Any of a number of problems, primarily with the lower or lumbar region of the vertebrae, that cause mild to severe discomfort; the most frequent complaint heard by doctors and the greatest cause of absenteeism at work; may be inherited or caused by a "slipped disk," poor posture, sciatica, lumbago, spondylitis, osteoarthritis, or rheumatoid arthritis; can often be treated with specific exercises.

backstroke

A swimming stroke executed while lying on the back; the arms are placed in the water behind the head and swept toward the thighs; coordinated with a flutter kick.

backward bend

An exercise performed from a kneeling position, intended to strengthen the abdominal muscles. The trunk is lowered slowly backward until the hands touch the floor behind the back; the exercise is completed when the trunk is returned to the original upright position.

badminton

A racquet game played on a 44' x 17' court with a net that is 61" high; two or four players volley a shuttlecock (usually a feathered object with a cork or plastic base; also called a bird) over the net with 26" long racquets; points are scored when the bird hits the ground or falls outside the playing area.

balance beam

A 4" wide wooden beam 30" off the floor designed for use in gymnastic exercises; beam may be a few inches off the floor for practice and for beginners.

balanced diet

Consists of appropriate amounts of food from the basic four food groups—dairy products; meat, fish, and poultry; vegetables and fruits; breads and cereals—to meet the needs of the body for carbohydrates, fats, proteins, vitamins, and minerals; amounts are calculated by age and weight (see *Basic Four Food Groups*); daily food consumption for an adult should include at least four servings of grain and cereal products, four or more servings of a variety of fruits and vegetables, two servings of dairy products, and two servings of meat, fish, or poultry.

ballistic stretching

Regular stretching exercises that are used to loosen the muscles but are performed more rapidly than ordinary stretching routines (see *stretching exercises*).

barbell

Any of a number of weight lifting implements that feature a bar with weights attached to either end; the bar measures anywhere from 36 to 72 inches; the weights are attached to and kept in place on the bar by means of collars that fasten at the end of the bar on the inside and outside of the weights; the weights can be made of iron or a cement-like material covered with plastic; weights come in sizes that range from ½ pound to 100 or more pounds (see *Nautilus* and *Universal*).

basal metabolic rate

The amount of energy required to maintain an organism at complete rest. It is measured in humans by the heat given off per unit of time and varies from person to person depending on height, weight, body type, and genetics. It is also called BMR; BMR is used to calculate how many calories a person should consume per day. To maintain weight, the average male needs 1,500 to 2,000 calories per day and the average female needs 1,200 to 1,500. BMR does not include the additional energy expenditure of exercise.

base

The amount of exercise it takes to provide a solid foundation of training to sustain the extra exertion of competition; in some forms of exercise, i.e., running, this base may take several years to acquire.

Basic Four Food Groups

The groupings of food that are essential to health and well-being; U.S. government nutritionists have identified these as the dairy group, the meat group, the vegetable and fruit group, and the bread and cereal group. Daily recommended servings for adults are: milk—two or more glasses, or servings of cheese, yogurt, ice cream, or other milk products; meat—two or more servings of meat, fish, poultry, or eggs; vegetables— four or more servings; breads and cereals—four or more servings (see *balanced diet*).

basket hang

An exercise intended to strengthen the abdominal muscles that is performed by suspending the body from a horizontal bar with the arms extended full length and the palms facing in; the knees are then flexed upward toward the chest, held, then lowered to the extended position.

belt vibrator

Motor-driven machines that vibrate the body with a belt that is attached to a cam-shaped wheel; usually used around the waist or the buttocks; intended to slim the area being vibrated; they are not useful for physical fitness.

bench press

A weight-lifting exercise performed from the supine position on a bench specifically designed for weight lifting (similar in size to a piano bench); the barbell is pressed straight upward until the arms are fully extended; the weight is then lowered to the starting position on or just above the chest; for full range of movement, begin the exercise with elbows below the plane of the bench; strengthens the chest and triceps muscles (see *dumbell press*).

bent-arm pullover

An exercise performed from the supine position; the barbell or dumbbell is pulled from behind the head to a position over the chest while keeping the elbows bent; the weight is lowered to the starting position to complete the exercise; strengthens the chest and triceps muscles.

bent-knee sit-up

A sit-up exercise performed from the prone position with knees bent, hands laced behind the head, and knees flexed so that the feet are flat on the floor; the trunk is curled upward until the elbows touch the knees and then lowered slowly back to the floor; strengthens the abdominal muscles; considered more beneficial than sit-up with legs extended because less pressure is placed on the lower back and more on the abdomen.

bent-over row

An exercise performed by bending at the waist and picking up the barbell or dumbbell from the floor; while remaining bent over at the waist, the weight is raised to the chest and then lowered back to the floor; the knees are kept straight throughout the exercise; strengthens both the chest and shoulder muscles.

beta-endorphin

A morphine-like chemical released by the body naturally during strenuous exercise that is said to cause a euphoric feeling; thought to be a cause of "runner's high," it originates in the pituitary gland and flows into the bloodstream (see *runner's high*).

biceps

The large flexor muscle on the front of the upper arm; flexes the elbow joint. The large flexor muscle on the back of the upper leg.

bicycle

An exercise performed from the supine position with the knees flexed to the chest; the pelvis is raised from the floor and held with the hands braced against the lower back; large circles are described by alternating the legs in a bicycling movement; strengthens the abdominals.

bicycling

The act of riding a bicycle; can be done for both exercise and pleasure; if used for aerobic exercise, pedaling must be continuous and performed against resistance, i.e., riding uphill or in high gear (see *stationary bicycle*).

biotin

A vitamin necessary for the formation of fatty acids and the release of energy from carbohydrates; found in egg yolk, liver, kidneys, dark green vegetables, and green beans.

blister

A condition that results when continuous rubbing of the skin damages underlying tissues, causing body fluids to accumulate and create a sensitive, liquid-filled swelling; at one time or another, blisters are an almost inevitable consequence of physical activity and can be serious if they become infected; when skin toughens, they are no longer a problem.

blood doping

The removal and subsequent reinfusion of blood for the purpose of temporarily increasing blood volume and the number of red blood cells; a controversial practice used by some athletes in the last stages of training; advocates say the practice improves performance; a technique used only by competitive athletes.

blood ejection velocity

The stroke volume of the heart; the speed with which the blood is forced from the heart.

blood glucose

The level of sugar in the blood (see *glucose*).

blood pressure

The driving force that moves blood through the circulatory system; normal blood pressure is approximately 120/80; systolic pressure (the higher number) is recorded when blood is ejected into the arteries; diastolic pressure (the lower number) is recorded when the blood drains from the arteries; physical training does not normally affect the resting blood pressure in younger people, but in those over 30 the resting blood pressure can be significantly reduced with training.

blood sugar

The simple sugar released from the liver into the bloodstream which nourishes all the body's cells; an adequate blood sugar level is vital for energy, alertness, general well-being; the average level of blood sugar is 60 to 100 milligrams for every 100 milliliters of blood, or less than six grams (¼ ounce) in a person weighing 140 pounds.

blood volume

The amount of blood in the body; for men, the average is 5 to 6 liters and for women, the average is 4 to 4.5 liters; physical training can result in a small increased blood volume; most of this increase is in the amount of plasma rather than an increase in actual red-cell volume; volume is important to the oxygen transport system during exercise.

bodybuilding

Exercise activity that uses weights or resistance machines to develop muscular strength and definition; used by athletes in all sports to develop strength for their particular sport; references to bodybuilding date back more than 2,000 years on a worldwide basis; professional bodybuilders compete in contests for money and prizes (see *Mr. America*).

body composition

The component parts of the body; commonly refers to fat and muscle weight (lean body mass); bodies with less fat have more lean body mass.

body contouring

A combination of diet and exercise; a euphemism used by health clubs and spas in place of diet and exercise.

body dynamics

Another term for aerobic movement (see *aerobic dancing*).

body temperature

The normal temperature of the body, which is usually 98.6°; when exercising, body temperature rises a degree or more.

body weight

The total weight of the body as measured on a scale.

bomb calorimeter

A device for measuring the calories in a specific amount of food. Food samples are placed in an insulated metal container along with a measured amount of oxygen. The bomb is placed in a water chamber with a measured amount of water and the sample is ignited electrically and burned. The heat of the burning raises the water temperature and the amount of temperature increase is the measure of calories in the food product.

bone

The dense, semirigid, porous, calcified connective tissue of the skeleton in most vertebrates.

bone bruise

Bleeding under the outside covering of the bone; can be caused by a blow to the affected area or is often the result of strenuous exercise; may be painful but usually disappears in a few days.

bone chip

A small portion of bone loosened from the main bone by injury or excessive use; can be treated with drugs or surgery.

bonking

A slang term for a condition that occurs when the body runs out of liver glycogen, which causes the blood sugar level to drop and the brain to function poorly; symptoms are dizziness, poor coordination, cold sweats, and confusion; liver glycogen can be replaced by eating foods high in potassium like bananas, but almost any food will do (see *the wall*).

born athlete

That mythical person who is born with the qualities of strength, speed, endurance, and skill that make for outstanding performance. It is mythical because dedication and training are also absolute necessities for any athlete.

Boston Marathon

The oldest and best known of the marathons run in this country, held every April. In order to enter, it is necessary to meet qualifying times in a given age group.

bradycardia

A decreased or slowed heart rate.

breast

The ventral or front surface of the upper body extending from the neck to the abdomen.

breastbone

See *sternum*.

breast stroke

A swimming stroke in which the swimmer lies face down in the water and extends his arms in front of his head, then sweeps them both back laterally under the surface of the water while performing a whip kick; a whole body exercise, but especially good for the shoulders and arms.

bulge

A protruding part; an outward curve or a swelling; can be caused by muscular development, fat, or swelling.

bulimarexia

The practice of eating large quantities of food and then forcing the body to purge itself either by taking laxatives or inducing vomiting; related to anorexia in that the desire of both the anorexic and the bulimarexic is to be thin (see *anorexia*).

bursa

A saclike body cavity, especially one located between joints or at points of friction between body parts that serves to cushion the moving parts of a joint.

bursitis

An inflammation of fluid-filled sacs (bursae) that cushion the moving parts of a joint; found especially at the shoulder, elbow, and knee joints and a common problem among athletes; a type of arthritis but more easily controlled through draining and medication.

butterfly

A swimming stroke in which the swimmer lies face down in the water and rapidly brings the arms out of the water to the sides and then over the head while arching the back and performing a flutter kick; a good all-body exercise.

buttock

Either of the two rounded parts of the rump (see *gluteus*).

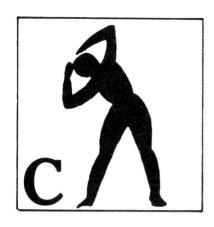

cable-tension test

A method of measuring strength of the skeletal muscles; originally consisted of a large wooden frame supported by uprights with handles attached to a crossbar that moved a weight; measured grip strength, pulling power of arm muscles, lifting power of back muscles; during World War II the Army Air Force used a similar but improved system in use today made of airplane cables and springs to test the strength of orthopedically disabled patients; 38 tests were constructed involving movements of the finger, thumb, wrist, forearm, elbow, shoulder, neck, trunk, hip, knee, and ankle; valuable in determining relative strength, particularly in physical rehabilitation.

caffeine

A stimulant derived from coffee, tea, and kola nuts, which is also a diuretic; said to improve performance if taken immediately before sporting events.

calcification

Impregnation with calcium or calcium salts, as with calcium carbonate; hardening occurs by such impregnation; usually affects joints that are used excessively, as the knees in long-distance running; can be treated with medication.

calcium

A metallic element; a basic component of bone, shells, and leaves; makes up approximately 85% of the mineral matter of bones.

calf

The fleshy, muscular part of the back of the leg between the knee and ankle.

calisthenics

Nonaerobic exercises based on gymnastics; primarily a series of stretching and jumping movements, designed to build muscular strength, endurance, and coordination; used by athletic teams and the armed forces for physical training; will increase endurance and strength if performed vigorously on a regular basis.

callus

A hardening of the skin created by repeated rubbing; common on the hands and feet of athletes.

caloric cost

The heat lost during all activity; physical activity requires energy for its performance; a convenient way of measuring the energy used is by determination of the oxygen consumed; that metabolic cost is expressed in calories per hour; e.g., the energy needs of a person sitting quietly have been calculated at 72 cal/hr.; during hard exercise, this calorie use may be increased 20 fold; one hour of running uses approximately 600 calories.

calorie

A unit of heat; the amount of heat required to raise the temperature of 1 kilogram of water by 1 degree centigrade; commonly used to express the energy-producing value of food; also called kilocalorie.

calorie count

The amount of food energy in a portion of food; e.g., one average apple contains 80 calories; a bowl of cornflakes has 95 calories, etc.

Cameron Heartometer

An instrument for evaluation of cardiovascular fitness; makes a recording of the pulse wave on a circular graph; used for fitness testing.

capillaries

Small vessels in a fine network located between arteries and veins throughout the body; capillaries enlarge slightly with exercise.

carbohydrate

A chemical compound containing carbon, hydrogen, and oxygen; important carbohydrates are starches, celluloses, and sugars; one of the three basic foods or macronutrients galong with fats and proteins.

carbohydrate loading

The practice of eating quantities of carbohydrate-heavy food prior to an endurance event; based on the theory that the muscles will be able to store more energy in the form of glycogen if they are loaded two or three days prior to an event; must be preceded by a carbohydrate-sparing diet and heavy exercise for two or three days; preferred foods include pasta, potatoes, bread, rice, and beans; also called carbohydrate packing.

cardiac arrest

The abrupt stoppage of the heart; commonly called a heart attack (see *heart attack*).

cardiac hypertrophy

An increase in the size of the heart; thought to result from athletic training; also called enlarged heart; a natural result of prolonged training; not considered dangerous.

cardiac muscle

The heart muscle; one of the three types of muscles in the body; can be developed by exercise.

cardiac output

The amount of blood pumped in one minute by either the left or right ventricle of the heart; the product of the heart rate and stroke volume.

cardiologist

A physician who specializes in the diagnosis and treatment of diseases of the heart.

cardio-respiratory

Pertains to the circulatory and respiratory systems; benefits from physical training of sufficient intensity.

cardiovascular system

The term used to describe the heart and the blood vessel system. The system benefits from physical training of sufficient intensity.

carotene

A hydrocarbon that is converted to Vitamin A in the liver; sources include yellow vegetables such as carrots, pumpkin, winter squash, and yams.

carotid

The large arteries on either side of the neck that carry blood to the head; can be used for taking the pulse.

carpus

The wrist; the eight bones between the forearm and the hand.

catabolism

A destructive phase of metabolism that results in the breakdown of complex material in the body.

cell

A small protoplasmic mass; the base unit of tissue.

cellular aging

Refers to the replacement of active tissue, such as muscle, by metabolically less active fat and connective tissue fibers.

cellulite

The name given to the fatty deposits that appear primarily on women's bodies as ripples on the thighs and buttocks; often treated differently than fat with special creams, sponges, and fad diets, but weight loss and the subsequent reduction in body fat is the only way to reduce cellulite.

center of gravity

A balance point; located in the area of the pelvis in humans; knowledge of the body's center of gravity is important for

athletes involved in such activities as gymnastics, high jumping, and pole vaulting.

central nervous system (CNS)

The portion of the nervous system consisting of the brain and
spinal cord; responsible for integrating all the various tissues
and systems of the body into a smoothly operating unit that
functions automatically; the information center of the body;
controls the body's muscular system—fine and gross motor
control.

cerebellum

The part of the brain responsible for the regulation and coordination of most voluntary muscular movement.

charley horse

A severe cramp usually in the upper thigh that can come from
a fall, a sharp blow, or overstretching a muscle or tendon;
origin of term unknown.

cheating

In weight lifting, the use of other muscles or muscle groups to
assist with an exercise in order to permit the handling of
greater poundage; the use of muscles not otherwise involved
in the exercise and often combined with the momentum of the
moving weight to give added leverage; usually used when the
muscles are tired; in dieting, the sneaking of food between
meals or in excess of the amounts prescribed in the diet.

chest pain

Pain in parts of the chest that may have a variety of causes;
some causes such as indigestion are relatively harmless; pain
may be caused or aggravated by exercise, muscle soreness,
inflammation of the rib cartilage, rib fracture or poor breathing;
serious chest pains may be an indication of heart trouble; also
called angina (see *angina pectoris*).

chinning bar

A bar suspended 7 to 9 feet above the floor that is used for
chinning exercises (see *chin-up*).

chin-up

An exercise performed with the body suspended from a horizontal bar with palms facing in; the body is pulled up until chin is over the bar, then lowered slowly; can also be performed with the palms facing out but is more difficult in that position; strengthens shoulder, forearms, and biceps muscles; also called pull-ups.

chiropractic

Manipulation of the spinal column and other bodily structures; a system of therapy in which disease is considered the result of neural malfunction.

chiropractor

A practitioner of chiropractics. Athletes often use chiropractors in the treatment of muscular problems.

cholesterol

An organic substance belonging to a group of crystalline or solid alcohols known as sterols; often called serum cholesterol; does not contain fatty acids but is often considered a member of the fat or lipid family; found in animal fats and oils, milk, and egg yolk. The liver is the primary regulator of body cholesterol. It serves as structural component of nerve tissue and sex hormones; it is essential to well-being but apparently dangerous in excessive quantity; high levels have been associated with coronary heart disease; exercise and a diet low in fats has been shown to lower the level of cholesterol.

chronograph

A clock that registers the time, usually of an athletic event.

chutes

The long, narrow lanes beyond the finish line at running races; usually designated by ropes or ribbons; designed to funnel competitors through the checking and timing process and into a rest area.

circuit training

A conditioning program consisting of a number of exercises performed at various stations; usually a given exercise is performed at a station within a specified time; the athlete then moves to the next station with its own particular exercise and specified time, and so on; a complete tour of the stations constitutes one circuit; a common method of weight training (see *weight training* and *progressive resistance exercise*).

circulation
The movement of blood through blood vessels as a result of the heart's pumping action.

circulatory-respiratory endurance
Moderate contractions of large muscle groups for relatively long periods of time during which maximal adjustments of the circulatory and respiratory systems are necessary, as in distance running and swimming; critical for the performance of events lasting 30 minutes or longer.

circulatory-respiratory system (C-R system)
The circulatory-respiratory system consists of the heart and lungs, the vessels supplying blood to all parts of the body, the oxygen carrying capacity of the blood, and the capillary system receiving the blood.

clavicle
The bone that links the sternum in the chest and the scapula, the flat, triangular bone (shoulder blade) that forms the back of the shoulder.

clean and jerk
See *Olympic lifting.*

coagulate
To cause the transformation of a liquid into a soft, semisolid or solid mass; to clot.

collagen
The main component of intercellular connective tissue.

collapse
Acute prostration or exhaustion; can result from excessive exercise, especially in hot weather.

collarbone

See *clavicle.*

coma

A state of profound unconsciousness; often the result of an injury.

competition

Vying with another or others for profit, prize, or position; rivalry; a driving and prevailing element in sports activities.

complexion

The natural color, texture, and appearance of the skin.

compulsive runner

A person who must run daily despite fatigue, weather, or injury: researchers at the University of Arizona found that compulsive runners exhibit anorexic tendencies, such as depression and anxiety, when unable to run.

concentric contraction

The shortening of muscles during physical activity, as in raising a weight (see *dynamic exercise* and *isotonic contraction*).

concentric movement

The type of movement that causes the muscles to shorten.

concussion

A jarring injury to the brain that impairs its normal function; can result in temporary or permanent damage.

conditioning

The process of training the body to a higher state of physical readiness or fitness.

congenital

Any physical trait existing at birth.

connective tissue

The tissue that binds together and is the support for the various structures of the body such as ligaments and tendons.

constrictor

In anatomy, a muscle that contracts or compresses a part or organ of the body.

contact lens

A thin plastic lens fitting over the cornea of the eye that usually eliminates the need for glasses; commonly used by athletes in all sports.

contort

To twist, wrench, or bend severely out of shape; some yoga asanas are contortions.

contractile

Capable of contracting or causing contraction.

contraction

The act of contracting; the shortening, and often thickening, of the muscle or muscles being used.

cool-down

A series of exercises designed to prevent too rapid cooling of the body and pooling of blood in the extremities: also to more rapidly dissipate the buildup of lactic acid in the system; exercises are much like the stretching movements used for warming up (see *warm-up* and *lactic acid*).

Cooper, Dr. Kenneth

Author and developer of aerobics, a method and series of exercises that is designed to develop cardiovascular fitness; in his system each exercise—running, rope skipping, swimming, biking—is given a point value based on the length of time of the exercise, its intensity, and the age of the exerciser; one of the pioneers in the physical fitness field.

coordination

The ability to control the movement of the muscles; used to refer to the ability of people, especially athletes, who have muscle harmony that enables them to perform difficult movements with relative ease.

copper

A mineral essential for health found in shellfish, liver, and vegetables such as dried peas, beans, and potatoes; also found in small amounts in other foods.

coronary collateral circulation

When a coronary artery supplying blood to a portion of the heart muscle is blocked, changes may occur in the coronary network that will enable blood from other arteries to reach the affected area of the myocardium; small new arteries may form a network to bypass the blocked or narrowed artery and promote collateral circulation; physical training has been shown to promote collaterals to compensate for compromised coronary circulation.

coronary heart disease.

Any of a variety of heart problems that affect the ability of the heart to function in a normal manner.

cortisone

A brain steroid active in carbohydrate metabolism; used to treat rheumatoid arthritis, adrenal insufficiency, certain allergies, diseases of connective tissue, and gout.

cramp

A sudden involuntary muscular contraction causing severe pain; often occurring in the leg or shoulder as a result of strain or chill; a temporary partial paralysis of habitually or excessively used muscles; in runners, sometimes called a "stitch" if it occurs in the side under the ribs near the diaphragm.

Crampton Blood Ptosis Test

A test for changes in heart rate and systolic blood pressure that occur upon standing after being in a reclining position.

crawl

A rapid swimming stroke in which the swimmer alternates overarm strokes while performing a flutter kick.

creatine

An organic acid similar to ATP found mainly in the muscle tissue of many vertebrates; acts with other phosphate compounds in muscular contraction; part of the energy production chain; produced by the body [see *adenosine triphosphate (ATP)*].

cross-country running

Running on nondesignated running areas, usually through terrain that features hills and flats; races vary in length from one and two miles to ten and twelve miles.

cross-country skiing

A sport and exercise performed with special skis, bindings, and shoes; requires less skill than downhill skiing but more endurance; done vigorously, it is one of the most effective methods of improving the circulatory-respiratory system.

C-R system

See *cardiorespiratory*.

Cureton, Thomas K.

Director of the Physical Fitness Institute, University of Illinois; internationally known investigator and practitioner of ways by which adult physical fitness can be improved and sustained; for more than 25 years he conducted and sponsored investigations on exercise regimens for adults.

curl

A barbell or dumbbell exercise performed in a standing position; the exerciser grasps the barbell or dumbbell with the arms by the sides and the palms facing out and slowly raises, or curls, the weight from the arms-extended position to the chest; the weight is then lowered to the starting position; strengthens the biceps (see *reverse curl*).

curl bar

An angled bar designed to increase the efficiency of the biceps curl exercise; the design of the bar places the hands and biceps in a position that is most conducive to performing the exercise.

curl-up

A sit-up performed by slowly curling up, starting with the head, then the shoulders, and finally curling the spine upward until a sitting position is reached; strengthens the abdominal muscles (see bent-knee sit-up).

C-V system

See *cardiovascular system*.

cycle

A time interval in which a regularly repeated event or sequence of events occurs; a single, complete execution of a periodically repeated function such as a cycle of exercises in which a number of different muscles are brought into play.

cycling

The act of riding either a stationary or a moving bicycle.

cytoplasm

A substance within the cell that contains a number of formed and dissolved elements, including enzymes that support the anaerobic metabolic processes of the cell.

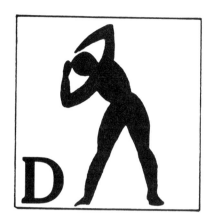

dead lift
See stiff-legged dead lift.

dead weight
The unrelieved weight of a heavy, motionless mass; the weight of a barbell is dead weight.

debilitate
To make feeble, enervate.

decalcify
To remove calcium from bones or teeth.

deep knee bend
An exercise performed by spreading the feet and lowering the body into a squatting position with the thighs parallel to the floor and the back straight.

dehydration
The condition resulting from excessive loss of body water caused by sweating; dangerous and sometimes fatal during exercise or athletic competitions.

DeLorme, Thomas L., and Watkins, Arthur L.
Credited with developing one of the first systematic isotonic weight training programs; originally designed for rehabilitation of veterans of World War II; refined the concept of repetition maximum, or RM, the maximal load a muscle or a muscle

group can lift a given number of times before fatiguing (see *repetition maximum* and *isotonic contraction*).

deltoid

The triangular muscle on the point of the shoulder and covering the shoulder; raises the arm from the side.

delts

A slang term used by bodybuilders and other athletes for the deltoid muscles (see *deltoid*).

De Mar, Clarence

Premier distance runner who entered 34 Boston Marathons from 1930 to 1965 and won seven; ran more than 1,000 races in his career, including 100 marathons; ran his last race at the age of 69.

depletion

A method of endurance training based on the theory that the muscles will learn to store more glycogen if the glycogen supply is almost completely used up (or depleted); it takes two or three extended workouts to deplete the muscles, depending on the condition of the exerciser; muscle aches and lack of coordination indicate a state of depletion; the opposite of carbohydrate loading (see *carbohydrate loading*).

derriere

The buttocks.

desirable weight

Weight guidelines based on averages established by insurance actuaries; determined by height and estimated body frame—small, medium, or large; useful only as a general guide.

detraining

The practice of tapering off following strenuous exercise; usually refers to the period just before an athletic event such as a long-distance race, when the runner cuts back on training time to allow the body to rest and recuperate.

develop

To expand or realize potentialities; bring gradually to a fuller, greater, or better state; also refers to muscular development and the development of cardiovascular fitness.

dexterity

Skill in the use of the hands or body; coordination.

dextrose

A sugar found in animal and plant tissue; can be derived synthetically from starch; also called corn sugar and dextroglucose (see *glucose*).

diastolic surge amplitude

The measurement of the sharp drop in systolic amplitude that occurs as the resistance in the arteries pushes back and closes the aortic valve of the heart; when the aortic valve closes, a recoil is transmitted back to the arteries, causing a secondary wave identified as diastolic surge amplitude, used in determining the health of the heart (see *systolic amplitude*).

diastolic wave

On a heartometer it represents the resting phase of the heart (see *Cameron Heartometer*).

diet

The usual food and drink of a person or animal; an organism's daily sustenance; a regulated selection of foods, especially as prescribed by a doctor for gaining or losing weight or for other medical reasons such as diabetes or high blood pressure.

dietary goals

Refers to the ideal diet; the type of diet recommended for health and nutrition for the average American by the Department of Agriculture, consisting of 58% carbohydrates, 30% fat, and 12% protein.

digestion

The bodily process by which foodstuffs are decomposed into simple, assimilable substances.

digestive system

The alimentary canal together with accessory glands including the salivary glands, liver, and pancreas; regarded as an integrated system responsible for food digestion.

digital watch

A faceless watch that displays the time with numbers, rather than hands; usually has stopwatch function that allows it to be used for timing sports events including races; popular with runners and other exercisers for timing workouts.

dip

An exercise performed with the body suspended between two parallel bars or chairs with the feet off the floor and the arms supporting the body; the body is lowered as far as possible using only the arms and then pressed back to the starting position; strengthens the deltoids and triceps.

disable

To weaken or destroy normal physical or mental abilities; to cripple.

disease

An abnormal condition of an organism or part of an organism especially as a consequence of infection, inherent weakness, or environmental stress; impairs normal physiological functioning.

distance running

The practice of running and preparing to run long distances such as the marathon (see *long slow distance*).

double-jointed

Having particularly flexible joints permitting connected parts, such as limbs or fingers, to be bent at unusual angles.

double-leg raise

An exercise performed from the supine position; the legs are raised to 90° and lowered slowly to starting position; strengthens the abdominal muscles (see *leg raise*).

downhill running

A method of training that involves practice running downhill;

thought to increase the speed of the firing of muscle fibers and therefore running speed over a period of time.

duck waddle

An exercise that is performed from the squatting position; the exerciser moves forward and backward while in that position, much like a duck waddles while walking; increases overall leg strength.

dumbbell

A short version of the barbell; the bar is 8· to 14 inches long and has collars for securing the weights; designed for use with one hand; may be made of one piece of molded iron, plastic, or chrome.

dumbbell press

An exercise performed from a standing, sitting, or prone position with a dumbbell in each hand; performed by pressing the weight up from the chest or shoulders until the arms are fully extended; may be done simultaneously or alternately; strengthens the deltoids and triceps (see *bench press*).

dumbbell swing

An exercise performed in the standing position with legs spread more than shoulder width by swinging a dumbbell in an arc from over the head until it passes between legs; strengthens the quadriceps, hamstrings, and gluteus maximus muscles.

duration

The length of time set aside for exercise or the length of time it takes to complete a given set of exercises; duration is closely linked to intensity and frequency of exercise (see *intensity* and *frequency*).

dynamic

Involving movement, as in movement of the muscles in exercise.

dynamic contraction

See *dynamic exercise* and *isotonics*.

dynamic exercise

Raising and lowering a load, such as a weight, a given number of times; involves contraction of the muscles; also called isotonic exercise.

Dynamic Tension

The trademark name of an isometric-like exercise program developed by Charles Atlas; involves pitting one set of muscles against another, but with some movement against the resistance (see *Atlas, Charles*).

dynamometer

Instrument used for measuring muscle strength; measures strength index (SI) and physical fitness index (PFI); SI is gross score of seven test items; PFI is a relative strength score that compares the SI to a norm for the individual's sex, age, and weight; dynamometer measures left and right hand grips, back and leg lifts, pull-ups, bar push-ups, and lung capacity.

dysmenorrhea

Lower abdominal pains or cramps during the menstrual period; often accompanied by headache, backache, leg ache, breast fullness or tenderness, abdominal swelling, or nausea; occurs most commonly just before or at the beginning of the menstrual flow and usually ceases when the flow is established; mineral supplements of calcium and magnesium along with regular exercise may lessen symptoms.

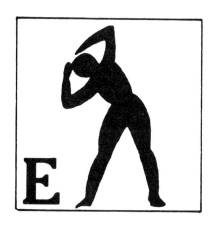

easy days

The days of an exercise routine that are relatively less strenuous than other days; most exercise schedules alternate easy days with workouts that require less energy output and hard days that require higher energy expenditure; easy days allow the body to recover between bouts of hard work and help prevent injury and undue fatigue.

eccentric contraction

Muscular contraction in which the muscle lengthens while developing tension (see *negative work*).

ectomorph

A somatotype; a person with a body type characterized by leanness, small bones, thin muscles, little fat, and linear structure; the long-distance runner is often an example of a person with ectomorphic qualities; other body types are mesomorph and endomorph.

efferent nerve

The motor nerve that conveys information from the central nervous system to organs such as glands and muscles.

elbow tendonitis

Inflammation causing tendon fibers to swell; also called tennis elbow; painful but pain lessens with activity; a common problem in athletics; tendonitis occurs in other areas of the body as well.

electrocardiogram (EKG)

A device used to record the electrical impulses that traverse the heart.

electrolyte

A substance that ionizes in solution, such as salt, and is capable of conducting an electrical current; vital for metabolism; must be replaced with liquid during and after exercise.

electromyography

The electromyograph is an instrument designed to pick up, amplify, and record electrical discharges created when muscles contract; useful for determining which muscles are involved in an exercise or body movement.

elongate

To lengthen or extend; to grow in length as the muscle in the extended portion of an exercise.

enarthrosis

A ball-and-socket joint, as in the hip.

endocardium

The thin membrane that lines the interior of the heart.

endocrine gland

Any of the ductless glands, such as the thyroid or andrenal glands, the secretions of which pass directly into the bloodstream from the cells of the gland; each gland manufactures its own material with specific chemical properties.

endomesomorph

A somatotype; a person with a body type that combines the tendency toward roundness of the endomorph and the heavy, hard, rectangular physique of a mesomorph.

endomorph

A somatotype; a person with a body type characterized by roundness often tending toward fat (see *ectomorph* and *mesomorph*).

endomysium

The connective tissue that surrounds a muscle fiber.

endurance

The ability of the muscles to perform work over a given period of time.

endurance training

A form of conditioning designed to increase aerobic capacity and endurance performance; usually consists of graduated and progressively more taxing bouts of exercise; necessary for events lasting more than 30 minutes (see *aerobic*).

energy

The capacity or ability to perform work.

energy balance

The balance that results when caloric expenditure equals caloric intake; e.g., when the daily energy (food) intake equals 2,500 calories and the daily expenditure of calories (basal metabolic rate plus calories consumed in work and exercise) equals 2,500 there is an energy balance.

enlarged heart

See *cardiac hypertrophy*.

enzyme

A protein compound that speeds up chemical reactions.

epicardium

The inner layer of the pericardium that is in actual contact with the heart (see *pericardium*).

epidermis

The outer, protective, nonvascular layer of the skin.

epilepsy

A nervous disorder characterized by recurring attacks of motor, sensory, or psychic malfunction with or without unconsciousness or convulsive movements.

epinephrine

Chemical name for adrenaline (see *adrenaline*).

equilibrium

Any condition resulting in a stable, balanced, or unchanging system; balance, which is important in athletic performance.

ERG

The trademark name of a drink containing a mixture of water, potassium, and salt designed to replace body fluids lost through sweat during exercise.

ergograph

Instrument used to measure the strength of elbow and shoulder flexion muscles; provides means for lifting and lowering a load of a given weight at a prescribed cadence; strength is measured by a repetition meter and a distance meter.

ergometer

A device attached to a treadmill or stationary bicycle, used for measuring the physiological effects of exercise; actually measures the amount of work or energy used in a specific test performed over a period of time and against resistance. It is the most accurate measure of energy consumption.

exercise

Any activity that requires physical or mental exertion, especially when performed to develop or maintain fitness; although most movement qualifies, it has come to mean more vigorous activity whose purpose is to raise the pulse and heart rate.

exercise stress test

A test to determine the ability of an individual to exercise with safety; conducted on a bicycle ergometer or a treadmill with adjustable grade; measurements taken include heart and pulse rate, blood pressure, and oxygen consumption; recommended for people over 35 who are beginning to exercise after having been sedentary.

exercise wheel

An exercise aid that consists of an axle and wheel; from a

kneeling position, the exerciser rolls the wheel away from and back toward the body; considered to be of minimum physical benefit.

Exer-Genie

The trademark name of a machine that provides constant resistance to the force exerted against it; after the machine is set, equal pressure is applied for the duration of the exercise movement.

exertion

The act of exerting energy, especially a strenuous effort.

exhale

To breathe out.

exhaustion

The state of being worn out completely; can result from vigorous exercise; not dangerous if sufficient time is allowed for recovery.

expanders

Any of a number of pieces of resistance equipment designed to strengthen muscles, tendons, and ligaments; compact and useful for training at home; made with rubber expansion bands, metal springs, and pneumatic tubes that provide isokinetic exercise, where the resistance increases as muscle effort is increased (see *isokinetic exercise*).

extensile

Capable of being stretched out.

external oblique

See *abdominal muscles*.

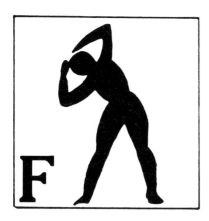

faint

An abrupt, usually brief loss of consciousness, generally associated with failure of normal blood circulation; sometimes occurs during or following exercise in hot weather.

fanny pack

A specially designed bag for hiking or running that is attached at the waist and is fastened with a belt; can hold small quantities and sits just over the buttocks so as not to impede arm and leg movement.

fartlek

A method of training that involves running a variety of distances at different speeds during one workout; could also be applied to biking, skiing, swimming (see *speed play*).

fascia

The strong, thick fibrous sheets that surround and support all the tissue in the body including muscles, tendons, joints, nerves, blood vessels, and organs; fascias absorb some of the pressure on these areas.

fasciculus

The largest subunit of skeletal muscle; muscle fibers in a fasciculus (plural: fasciculi) may number from one to over one hundred.

fast

To abstain from eating all or certain foods for a given period of time; a method of dieting that forces quick weight loss; rarely recommended by doctors because of the dangers of dehydration and vitamin deficiency.

fast foods

Any of a wide variety of foods, including hamburgers, chicken, tacos, etc., that are prepared quickly at home or sold at special restaurants or stands; often fried or high in sodium; not recommended for dieters or people with hypertension (see *junk food*).

fast twitch fibers

White muscle fibers that are considered fast-acting and are characterized by fast contraction time; suited for high-power activities, they are more prevalent in athletes who participate in sports events like sprinting, which require speed more than endurance.

fat

A foodstuff containing glycerol and fatty acids; in the body: the soft tissue other than that making up the skeletal muscle mass and the viscera; any of various soft solid or semisolid organic compounds comprising the glyceride esters of fatty acids and associated phosphatides, sterols, alcohols, hydrocarbons, ketones, and related compounds; used for energy during prolonged exercise, especially distance running.

fat-free weight (FFW)

That portion of the body weight remaining when the weight of body fat is subtracted from the total body weight; mainly the weight of the skeletal muscle mass; measured by calipers or immersion in special water tanks.

fatigue

Physical or mental weariness or exhaustion resulting from physical exertion; the decreased capacity or complete inability of an organism or part of an organism to function normally because of excessive stimulation or prolonged exertion.

fatty

Containing fat; characteristic of fat.

feet stabilized

A term that refers to a position in any exercise where the feet are held down by a partner or by placing them under a fixed support; used in performing sit-ups with knees bent or straight and back hyperextension.

FFA

See *free fatty acid.*

FFW

See *fat-free weight.*

fiber

An indigestible carbohydrate in food, found in the cell walls of plants; fiber is the substance in food necessary for the normal passage of undigested food through the intestine; also referred to as "nature's broom."

fibrillation

Irregular and uncoordinated contractions of the heart.

fibula

The outer and smaller of two bones of the leg between the knee and the ankle; the continual pounding of long-distance running can cause stress fractures in this area (see *stress fracture* and *shin splints*).

fit

Physically sound; healthy; exhibiting the characteristics of physical fitness (see *fitness*).

fitness

Defined by the President's Council on Physical Fitness and Sports as: "the ability to carry out daily tasks with vigor and alertness, without undue fatigue, and with ample energy to enjoy leisure time pursuits and to meet unforeseen emergencies"; the three basic components of fitness are muscular strength, muscular endurance, and circulatory-respiratory endurance; other components include muscular power, agility, speed, and flexibility.

5BX Program
A progressive schedule of five calisthenic exercises for men and women developed by the Royal Canadian Air Force (see *Royal Canadian Air Force Plans for Physical Fitness*)

Fixx, James F.
Author of *The Complete Book of Running* and other books on running; widely credited with stimulating the interest in jogging in America that began in the mid-1970s.

flabby
Without firmness; loose and yielding to the touch; usually refers to someone out of shape, not fit.

flank
The section of flesh betwen the last rib and the hip; the side.

flat feet
Feet with an abnormal inward roll (see *pronated feet*).

flex
To bend the body; to contract a muscle.

flexed-arm hang
An exercise performed while hanging from a chinning bar with the arms in the flexed position; the position is held for several seconds; strengthens the biceps and shoulder muscles.

flexibility
The range of possible movement around a joint or a sequence of joints; e.g., the ability to swing the arm like a propeller shows a full range of motion and indicates flexibility of that joint and the muscles around it; flexibility is a specific rather than a general trait, i.e., some joints are more flexible than others.

flexor
A muscle that acts to flex a joint.

folic acid
A vitamin that assists in forming body proteins, genetic

material, and hemoglobin; found in liver, kidneys, dark green leafy vegetables, wheat germ, and brewer's yeast.

food energy

The amount of energy or calories available in an item of food; the number of calories consumed.

footing

A secure placement of the feet in standing or moving.

fracture

A break, rupture, or crack, as in bone or cartilage.

free fatty acid (FFA)

The usable form of triglycerides (see *triglycerides*).

freestyle

A swimming stroke, usually the crawl (see *Australian crawl*).

free weights

The term used for barbells and dumbbells; weights that are not connected to a machine.

French curl

A barbell exercise; performed either from the sitting position or lying on a bench; bending only at the elbows, the weight is lowered from the arms-extended position over the chest to the forehead and then back to the starting position; strengthens triceps (see *pulldown* and *triceps extension*).

frequency

The number of times per week an exercise or an exercise routine is performed; e.g., the recommended number (frequency) of weight training workouts is 3 to 4 per week; closely linked to duration and intensity (see *duration* and *intensity*).

fructose

One of the four 6-carbon sugars (others are glucose, galactose, and mannose); also known as fruit sugar; found in most fruits.

full squats

A deep-knee bend in which the thighs are lowered below a

position parallel with the floor; can be harmful to the knees if performed too frequently and with too much weight (see *deep-knee bends*).

functional isometrics

Isometric contractions performed with weights and with the use of a device called a power rack, from which weights are lifted, and against which weights are held (see *power rack*).

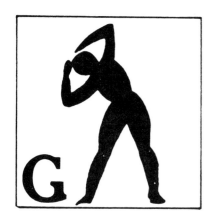

gastrocnemius
The muscle group that comprises the bulk of the calf of the leg.

Gatorade
The trademark name of a drink formulated to replace body fluids lost through sweat during exercise.

genetics
The biology of heredity; the study of the transmission and variation of the characteristics of organisms.

gland
An organ that extracts specific substances from the blood and concentrates or alters them for subsequent secretion.

glucose
A soluble sugar that is found in many foods, especially those high in carbohydrates (bread, grain products, potatoes), and is produced naturally in the body by the breakdown of dietary starch; one of the four 6-carbon sugars (see *fructose*); also known as dextrose, corn sugar, or grape sugar.

glutes
Slang term used by bodybuilders and other athletes to describe the gluteus maximus muscles in the buttocks.

gluteus
Any of three large muscles of the buttocks: gluteus maximus,

which extends to the thigh; gluteus medius, which rotates and adducts the thigh; gluteus minimus, which abducts the thigh (see *abduct* and *adduct*).

glycogen

The carbohydrate stored in the liver that provides the body with a reserve of energy. It is converted to glucose on demand of active muscles and is vital in endurance training and endurance races.

glycogen loading

An exercise-diet procedure that supposedly elevates muscle glycogen to concentrations two to three times normal; accomplished by first depleting the muscles of their glycogen by strenuous exercise and then "loading" or "packing" the muscles with glycogen by eating a diet rich in carbohydrates (see *carbohydrate loading* and *glycogen*).

glycogen sparing

The diminished utilization of glycogen that results when other fuels are available for activity; e.g., when fat is used for energy to a greater extent than usual, glycogen is spared; glycogen is thus available longer before ultimately being depleted; the glycogen supply is vital for endurance athletes (see *glycogen*).

goniometer

A device for testing the range of motion; consists of a 180° protractor with extended arms, which measures the rotation of the extremities; used to evaluate flexibility.

good morning

An exercise performed by bending at the waist with a barbell on the shoulders until the chest is parallel with the floor and returning to the standing position; strengthens the quadriceps, hamstrings, and gluteus maximus.

granola

Mixtures of variously processed grains with bits of dried fruit and nuts added, along with sweetener; originated in Swiss and German health spas in the early 1900s; has no added vitamins and minerals; supposed to be a "quick energy" snack.

gravity boot

A padded bootlike device with hooks that allows a person to hang upside down from a bar or a specially constructed frame; said to aid in blood circulation, improve posture, and reduce back problems; there is no research to support these claims.

groin ringworm

A red, sometimes flaky rash, often accompanied by ring-shaped markings in the groin area and the inner parts of the upper thighs; often contracted by athletes, it is caused by a fungus.

gymnasium

A room or building equipped for gymnastics and other sports; a modern gym may have weight-lifting equipment and machines, a swimming pool, sauna, steam room, running track, and other amenities.

gymnastics

Exercises, especially those performed with special apparatus in a gymnasium (see *parallel bars, rings, balance beam*).

gym shorts

See *running shorts*.

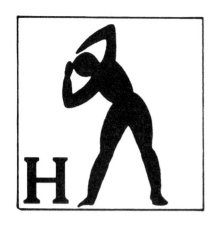

habit

A constant, often unconscious inclination to perform some act; acquired through frequent repetition; i.e., exercising daily.

hack squat

An exercise similar to the full squat, but with the barbell held in the arms-extended position behind the knees; strengthens the quadriceps (see *squat* and *deep-knee bends*).

half squat

An exercise performed by spreading the feet and lowering the body into a position that is halfway between a standing and a squatting position with the knees flexed and the back straight, puts less pressure on the knees than full squats (see *squat* and *deep-knee bends*).

hamstring pull

A relatively serious injury to one of the hamstring muscles; usually requires extended rest for healing; often results when quadriceps muscle is stronger than hamstring; warm-up and cooldown exercises can help prevent this injury (see *quadriceps*).

hamstrings

The three bulky muscles at the back of the thigh; they are the muscles that extend the thigh when the leg is flexed.

hand grip

A piece of exercise equipment, usually a strong spring with

two handles, that is designed to be placed in the palm of the hand and squeezed until the handles touch; increases strength in the fingers, wrists, and forearms; a rubber ball may be used for the same purpose.

hand weights

Light weights, like dumbbells, carried in the hands while exercising to add resistance; used by runners to help develop the muscles of the arms.

hard days

The days of a regular exercise routine that are relatively more strenuous than other days (see *easy days*).

Harvard Step Test

A fitness test performed by stepping up and down on a 20-inch bench 30 times per minute for five minutes; tests pulse rate recovery; similar tests are performed on lower benches or steps and for intervals of three to five minutes; gives an accurate reading of the ability to exercise at submaximal levels.

Hatha yoga

A type of yoga practiced as a preparation for the more meditative and intellectual schools of yoga; the initial step in the study of yoga; "yoga" means to join together or to yoke; the practice of the asana (postures or positions) of this type of yoga, its breathing patterns and purification techniques, is said to cause a gradual awareness and understanding of the creative and spiritual aspects that support the conscious mind and body (see *yoga*).

HDL

See *high density lipoprotein*.

headgear

A covering, such as a hat or helmet, for the head; protects against sports injuries and the sun.

health

Defined by the World Health Organization as "physical, mental, and social well-being"; not merely the absence of disease and infirmity.

health club
A private club that provides members with a variety of health-oriented activities that may include swimming, weight lifting, racquetball, squash, tennis, handball, aerobic exercise, steam and sauna baths; activities usually are supervised by trained personnel.

health food
Any of a wide variety of foods said to be valuable for health and fitness because of specific qualities that may include a high percentage of vitamins and minerals; often refers to items that are organically grown, i.e., without the use of artificial fertilizers or chemicals; found in stores that specialize in these products.

health spa
See *spa*.

heart
The hollow, muscular organ in vertebrates that pumps blood received from the veins into the arteries and supplies the entire circulatory system with it; weighs approximately one pound and is 5″ long by 3½″ wide; consists of right and left atrium and right and left ventricle; beats about 40 million times a year; pumps 2,000 gallons of blood a day.

heart attack
The condition or instance of heart failure; any seizure or abnormal heart functioning (see *cardiac arrest*).

heart block
A heart irregularity; a change in the rhythm of the heart resulting in decreased cardiac output.

heartburn
A burning sensation in the lower end of the esophagus; often caused by overeating or eating spicy food.

heart failure
A condition in which the heart cannot pump blood at a rate or volume adequate to sustain life.

heart-lung system

See *cardio-respiratory*.

heart murmur

An abnormal murmuring sound heard through the chest wall, which can be congenital; individuals with known heart murmurs should see a physician before beginning an exercise program.

heartograph

A graph made by a heartometer that shows the strength of the heartbeat (see *Cameron Heartometer*).

heartometer

See *Cameron Heartometer.*

heart rate (HR)

The number of times the heart beats per minute; normal rate is approximately 70 beats per minute at rest.

heat cramp

A heat illness caused by prolonged exposure to environmental heat characterized by painful muscular contractions (spasms), heavy sweating, fatigue; normal body temperature continues; treatment includes immediate cooling of the body; can progress to heatstroke.

heat exhaustion

A heat illness caused by fatigue resulting from prolonged exposure to environmental heat characterized by extreme weakness, dizziness, nausea, profuse sweating, rapid pulse, and sometimes unconsciousness; normal body temperature continues; treatment includes immediate cooling of the body; can progress to heatstroke.

heat illness

Incapacitation from excessive environmental heat; less serious than heat exhaustion or heatstroke; treated by cooling the body.

heat production

The result of the breakdown of a given amount of glycogen or fat; can be measured as amount of heat produced or amount of oxygen consumed; consumption of one liter of oxygen with glycogen as the food fuel releases 5 kilocalories of heat; there is a direct relationship between oxygen consumption and energy and heat production in the body.

heat prostration

A heat illness characterized by cold, pale skin, and profuse sweating, which may be accompanied by weakness, dizziness, nausea, or blurred vision; results from the body's temporary inability to adjust its natural responses to heat; similar to heat exhaustion and less serious than heatstroke.

heat stress

The load imposed by environmental heat; evaluated by the degree to which various activities become difficult or impossible to perform in the heat; poses no risk to health.

heatstroke

A condition characterized by dry, hot skin, a sudden rise in body temperature to 105° or more, nausea, confusion, collapse, and sometimes death; caused by exposure to environmental heat; emergency treatment includes providing immediate cooling by any means available for this most dangerous heat illness.

Heavy Hands

Brand name for a high-tech hand weight (see *hand weights*).

heavy legs

A feeling that occurs in the legs during a long workout; usually denotes a depletion of glycogen.

heel

The rounded posterior portion of the foot under and behind the ankle.

heel and toe

See *race walker*.

heel raise

See *toe raise*.

heel spur

A small, extra piece of heel bone that sticks out where the plantar fascia attaches to the heel; may or may not cause pain (see *plantar fasciitis*).

hemal

Pertaining to the blood or blood vessels.

hematosis

Oxygenation of venous blood in the lungs.

hemoglobin

A complex compound found in red blood cells that contains 6% iron (heme) and 94% protein (globin); combines with oxygen and transports oxygen throughout the body.

heredity

The genetic transmission of characteristics by parents to their children; among these characteristics are muscle fiber type, aerobic capacity, and neuromuscular capacity.

high density lipoprotein (HDL)

The transport system that clears excess cholesterol from artery walls and returns it to the liver for excretion; helps prevent excess deposits of cholesterol; research indicates that exercise may increase the amount of HDL and have a positive effect on decreasing the accumulation of cholesterol on artery walls.

hiking

Walking, usually cross-country, for recreation and fitness.

hip

The laterally projecting prominence of the pelvis or pelvic region from the waist to the thigh.

hip roll

An exercise performed from the supine position; knees are flexed and pulled up to chest and body is rolled from side to side; contributes more to relaxation of the upper body than to strength, endurance, or aerobic capacity.

hitting the wall
See *the wall.*

hollow sprints
Running two sprints with a hollow period, or time of jogging or walking, between the two sprints.

holozoic
Obtaining nourishment by the ingestion of organic material.

horizontal bar
A flexible bar used in gymnastics; suspended 8′ 5″ from the floor and used for a variety of swings, circles, and turns.

hot tub
See *whirlpool bath.*

HR
See *heart rate.*

humerus
The long bone of the upper part of the arm extending from the shoulder to the elbow.

hydrostatic weight
Body weight obtained by a method for assessing body volume that uses the physical principle that a body immersed in fluid is acted on by a buoyancy force which is evidenced by a loss of weight equal to the weight of the displaced fluid; used when determination of exact lean body weight (muscle and bone) is desired; requires special equipment including a water tank.

hyperflexible
The ability to flex around joints to a greater degree than the average person.

hyperglycemia
The presence of an abnormally high concentration of glucose (sugar) in the blood; caused by the inability of the body to handle normal amounts of glucose; can result in diabetes; blood sugar can reach levels 20 times higher than normal (normal range is 0.1 to 0.2% by weight).

hyperinsulinism

The presence of abnormally high quantities of insulin in the blood; can result in hyperglycemia.

hyperkinesia

Excessive, often undirected, motion.

hypertension

High blood pressure (see *blood pressure*).

hyperthermia

Excessively high body temperature.

hypertrophy

The growth and increase in size of a muscle cell; bodybuilders are examples of extreme hypertrophy of the muscles.

hyperventilation

Excessive movement of air into and out of the lungs; caused by increased depth and frequency of breathing; related to large increases in carbon dioxide and lactic acid that accompany vigorous exercise; causes buzzing in the ears, tingling of extremities, and sometimes fainting.

hypervitaminosis

Any of a number of abnormal conditions in which the physiological effect of a vitamin is produced to an excessive degree by use of the vitamin.

hypoflexible

Abnormally restricted flexibility in the joints.

hypoglycemia

Abnormally low level of glucose (sugar) in the blood. Normal amounts of blood sugar are in the range of 0.1 to 0.2% by weight (see *hyperglycemia*).

hypothermia

A condition that develops when the body temperature falls below 98.6°; caused by the body's attempts to warm the skin by opening up the skin blood vessels; the first symptom is red skin; other symptoms include the inability to enunciate clearly, numb fingers, and shivering; can be caused by outdoor exercise in very cold weather; can prove fatal without medical attention.

hypothyroidism

Insufficient production of thyroid hormones (see *thyroid gland*).

hypotonic

Having less than normal tone or tension in the muscles.

hypoxia

Lack of adequate oxygen; occurs at high altitudes; caused by a decrease in the pressure of oxygen in the air; results in a decline in VO_2max; at altitudes above 5,000 feet, the decrease in VO_2 is about 3% per 1,000 feet; in well-trained athletes, the decline begins at 1,000 feet and continues at the rate of 2% per 1,000 feet of altitude; especially taxing for those participating in endurance events (see *maximum oxygen uptake*).

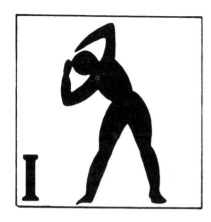

ideal weight

The weight that is optimal for a person's body type, height, and age; guidelines established by Metropolitan Life Insurance Co. and accepted by most doctors (see Appendix for chart).

ideal workout

The balanced method of exercise, which consists of three parts; a period of warm-up exercises to build up body heat, circulation, and respiration and to protect muscles and joints from strain by reducing their resistance to movement; various kinds of relatively strenuous exercises such as running, swimming, or bicycling; a period of tapering-off that emphasizes deep breathing, stretching, massage, and rest.

ileum

A portion of the small intestine.

ilium

The uppermost and widest of the three bones comprising one of the halves of the pelvis.

incapacity

Lack of strength or ability; disability; helplessness.

incline board

See *bench.*

incline press

An exercise; a bench press performed from an inclined board; strengthens the chest and triceps muscles (see *bench press*).

indigestion

Difficulty in digesting food; characterized by a burning sensation in the stomach or lower part of the esophagus and the
formation of gas in the stomach; also called heartburn; usually
relieved by taking antacids.

infarct

A dead area in an organ or tissue resulting from circulatory
blockage; e.g., myocardial infarction or heart attack.

ingest

To take in by swallowing.

injure

To cause harm or damage, to hurt.

innervate

To supply a bodily part with nerves; to stimulate a nerve or
bodily part.

intensity

The effort involved or applied to an exercise; e.g., running or
bicycling uphill is a more intense exercise than running or
bicycling on a flat surface; as intensity increases, duration
decreases; related to frequency and duration of exercise (see
frequency and *duration*).

internal oblique

See *abdominal muscles.*

international units (I.U.s)

The measure most often found in tables of recommended
amounts of vitamins and minerals; a single measure used to
describe the values of vitamin compounds.

interval training

A term applied to running; an exercise program in which the
body is subjected to short but repeated periods of work inter-
spersed with adequate periods of rest; useful for increasing
running speed; intervals may vary from activities lasting a few
seconds to several minutes; an interval workout might include
two runs of 220 yards with a one-minute period of walking or

jogging between runs, four runs of 440 yards with walking between, and so on; a variety of training modes can be used including jog-rest, jog-walk, slow jog-fast jog, and jog-sprint; allows the runner to increase total training time without undue stress.

intramuscular
Activity within a muscle.

intravascular
Activity within the blood vessels or lymphatics.

invigorate
To impart vigor, strength, or vitality.

iodine
A nonmetallic element of the halogen group; essential in small amounts in the diet (as in iodized salt) for the proper development and functioning of the thyroid gland.

isokinetic contraction
Muscular contraction executed at a constant speed and in such a fashion that the tension developed by the muscle while shortening is maximal over the full range of joint motion.

isokinetic exercise
The type of muscular exercise in which resistance is provided by friction, e.g., using an exercise bicycle that has adjustable tension; this controlled velocity of movement imposes continued maximum resistance on the contracting muscle or muscles.

isometric contraction
Muscular contraction without movement; occurs when the ends of the muscle are fixed in place so that significant increases in tension are produced without appreciable increases in length of the muscle; e.g., holding a weight at arm's length or trying to lift an immovable object; also called static contraction.

isotonic contraction
Muscular contraction in which the muscle shortens with varying tension while lifting a constant load; also referred to as

dynamic contraction and concentric contraction (see *dynamic contraction* and *concentric contraction*).

isotonics
Raising and lowering a load, such as a weight, a given number of times; sometimes called istonic exercise or dynamic training.

itching
A persistent irritation of the cutaneous tissues that causes an urge to scratch; often said to result from mild stimulation of pain receptors.

I.U.s
See *international units.*

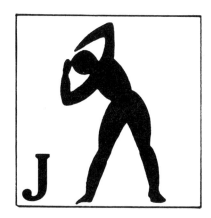

Jacuzzi
The trademark name of a whirlpool device that can be placed in the home bathtub (see *whirlpool baths*).

jargon
Terms or expression peculiar to a specific activity or field of interest; e.g., fitness jargon such as "p.r.," "reps," "fartlek," and "split time."

jock itch
A red, flaky rash in the groin or the inner part of the upper thigh usually the result of a fungus infection; aggravated by warm weather and sweating; can be treated with skin cream.

jockstrap
See *athletic supporter.*

jogger
See *treadmill.*

jogging
A generic term for all types of short- and long-distance running from very slow to very fast; commonly used to describe a slow run that is noncompetitive but is still fast enough to improve cardio-respiratory endurance; a slower form of running; more than 17 million Americans are said to jog on a regular basis.

joint
A point of connection between more or less movable parts, as between bones or segments in the leg.

judo

A form of the martial arts, formerly called jujitsu, that uses balance and leverage to overcome an opponent's size and strength; often used for physical training.

junk food

A variety of food items such as pizza, potato chips, soda pop, candy, and certain other fast foods and snacks that are generally high in calories and/or sugar and low in vitamins and minerals; can be nutritious as well; e.g., pretzels, hot dogs; these items also often contain abnormally high amounts of sodium; designated "junk foods" by the proponents of health foods; generally shunned by athletes and proponents of exercise and fitness.

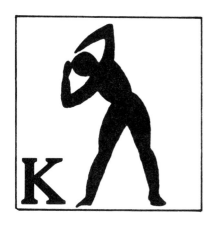

karate

A Japanese form of the martial arts; means empty-handed; an unarmed method of self-defense that stresses blows to strategic parts of the body; also used to develop fitness (see *martial arts*).

kcal

See *kilocalorie*.

ketone

An organic compound having a carbonyl group linking two carbon atoms.

ketosis

An abnormal increase of ketone bodies; the accumulation of toxic substances in the blood; can lead to kidney damage; a possible side effect of severe dieting or the carbohydrate-loading phase of training for long-distance running events; problem can be avoided or minimized by drinking large quantities of fluids.

kilocalorie (kcal)

The equivalent of 1,000 small calories; the accepted measure of food energy; however, "calorie" is the term in common use.

kilogram (kg.)

One thousand grams; 2.2 kilograms equals one pound.

kilometer

A distance that is the equivalent of 3/5 of a mile; used for measuring distance in races, e.g., a 10K is equal to 6.2 miles.

kinesia
Motion sickness.

kinesialgia
Pain caused by muscular activity.

kinesiology
The branch of science concerned with the study of muscles, muscle groups, and muscular movement.

kinesthesia
Sensory awareness of bodily movements such as muscular movements.

kinesthetic sense
Awareness of body position; also called kinesthesis.

kinetic energy
Energy associated with motion.

kinetics
The study of all aspects of motion and the relationship between motion and the forces that affect motion.

knee
The joint of the leg that connects the femur, tibia, and patella.

kneecap
A flat triangular bone on the front of the knee; the patella.

knee jerk
An involuntary kick of the lower leg that occurs when the tendon just below the kneecap is given a strong tap.

Kraus-Weber Test
A test of flexibility; starting from a standing position with the knees straight, exercisers must touch the floor with the fingertips and hold the position for 3 seconds.

kung fu
A form of the martial arts (see *martial arts*).

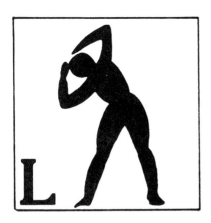

lacerate
To tear roughly or jaggedly.

laceration
A ragged or torn wound.

lactic acid
A fatiguing metabolite formed as a result of the incomplete breakdown of carbohydrate; usually occurs during endurance activities; causes muscles to ache.

lactic acid system
The system that produces lactic acid, one of the products left when sugar in the body is only partially broken down; an anaerobic energy system in which ATP is manufactured; high intensity efforts requiring one to three minutes to perform draw energy (ATP) primarily from this system; when lactic acid accumulates in the muscles and blood and reaches high levels, temporary muscle fatigue results; can be the cause of early fatigue during exercise; light exercise rather than complete rest is best for eliminating the accumulated lactic acid and returning the body to its pre-exercise state; also called alactic acid system.

LaLanne, Jack
One of the pioneers in the exercise field; had the first television exercise program in the 1950s; a highly trained man who uses calisthenics as the basis of his routines; operates health clubs in many cities; a tight-fitting jumpsuit is his trademark.

lap

One complete turn or circuit, especially of a running track or swimming pool.

lap time

The time it takes to complete one lap of a circuit.

lassitude

A feeling of profound weakness or fatigue; can result from overtraining.

lateral raise

An exercise performed with a dumbbell in each hand; the weights are raised from the sides until they reach shoulder height, then lowered to the starting position; strengthens the chest and the deltoids; can also be performed from the supine position.

latissimus dorsi

The broad muscles of the back behind the rib cage and attached to it at the mid-chest.

lat pulldown

See *pulldown.*

lats

A slang term used by bodybuilders and other athletes for the latissimus dorsi muscles that span the upper back.

lax

Not taut, firm or compact; slack.

layoff

See *reversibility.*

lean body mass

That portion of the body weight remaining when the weight of body fat is subtracted from the total body weight; mainly the weight of the skeletal muscle mass; also called fat-free weight.

lecithin

Any group of phosphatides found in all plant and animal

tissues; produced commercially from egg yolks, soybeans, and corn; used in the processing of foods, pharmaceuticals, cosmetics, paints and inks, and rubber and plastics; sold in granule, pill, and capsule form; not a vitamin; said to lower blood cholesterol levels and prevent heart disease, but this claim is not yet confirmed by scientific evidence.

leg curl
An exercise performed while lying on the stomach with the legs fully extended; the lower legs are curled up against resistance—a partner's hands or a machine designed for that purpose; strengthens the hamstrings and the gluteus maximus muscles.

leg extension
An exercise performed from the supine position with legs straight; knees are flexed to the chest, then extended slowly to starting position by sliding heels along surface.

leg lift
See *leg raise.*

leg press
An exercise performed lying on the back with the feet under a shelflike device that holds weights and slides up and down on parallel bars; as the legs are pressed upward the weights are raised; when the legs are returned to the starting position the weights are lowered; strengthens the quadriceps; also called leg extension. On Nautilus and other machines this exercise is done in the sitting position.

leg raise
An exercise performed form the supine position with the legs extended; legs are lifted without bending until they are at right angles with the body; may also be done one leg at a time; strengthens the abdominal muscles.

Leighton Flexometer
Instrument used to measure the range of motion of various joints throughout the body, including the trunk and extremities.

ligament

A sheet or band of tough, fibrous tissue that connects two or more bones at the joints, or supports an organ, fascia, or muscle.

lipid

Fat.

liposis

Excessive body fat.

lithe

Moving easily; supple; limber; flexible.

loin

The part of the side and back between the ribs and the pelvis.

long slow distance (LSD)

The practice of exercising for fitness or training for races, which involves running slowly for distances of up to 100 miles a week; slowly usually means at the rate of 8 to 9 minutes per mile.

loose-jointed

Having freely moving joints.

loose-limbed

Having freely moving limbs.

LSD

See *long slow distance.*

lumbago

A spasm of the muscles in the lumbar region of the back; can occur after exercise and can be severe enough to prevent the sufferer from standing; a cause of back pain.

lumbar

Relating to the loins or the region of the back and sides between the lowest ribs and the pelvis.

lymph

A slightly yellowish liquid circulated in the lymphatic vessels; bathes the tissues and carries away waste.

lymphatic system

The interconnected system of spaces and vessels between tissues and organs by which lymph is circulated throughout the body.

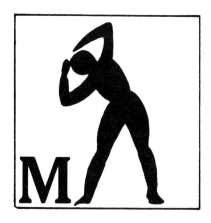

macronutrients

Carbohydrates, fats, and proteins.

marathon

A race of 26 miles, 385 yards; length of the race was determined by the distance from the battlefield at Marathon to Athens, Greece, the distance supposedly covered by the messenger Pheidippides, who brought news of the Greek victory over the Persians at Marathon and then collapsed and died; the most prominent of several hundred marathons in the U.S. every year are held in Boston and New York City.

marathon stone

A stone erected on the spot where Pheidippides delivered his message of victory from the battlefield at Marathon after running 26 miles, 385 yards; legend says he shouted, "Rejoice, we conquer," before dying of exhaustion; the 1,850-pound stone is stored at City University of New York.

martial arts

A term used to describe several Oriental methods of physical training, self-defense, and discipline; such forms as karate, jujitsu, T'ai Chi, judo, and others are included.

massage

The rubbing or kneading of various parts of the body to aid circulation and relax the muscles; used extensively by athletes and others for rehabilitation following injury.

mat

A cushioned covering for a hard surface, especially for exercise purposes; available in a variety of sizes and thicknesses; provides comfort and helps prevent injury.

mat burn

A skin abrasion resulting from falls to the mats covering the floor in exercise areas; generally harmless but should be protected against infection.

maximal oxygen consumption

The maximal rate at which oxygen can be consumed per minute, also called VO_2max; the power or capacity of the aerobic oxygen system.

maximum heart rate

The rate at which the heart can no longer meet the body's demand for oxygen and cannot beat any faster; the maximum rate can be figured by subtracting age from 220; e.g., a person 40 years old would have a maximum heart rate of 180; fitness exercises that force the heart rate up to 60 to 80% of maximum are considered adequate for improving or maintaining the cardiovascular system.

maximum oxygen uptake (VO_2 max)

The amount of oxygen metabolized by the body with the demands of a given workload; reflects the ability of the ventricles of the heart to put out an increased stroke volume; measures the upper limit of aerobic work capacity in man; the principal measure of improvement in circulatory-respiratory fitness.

McCurdy-Larson Test

The sitting diastolic blood pressure; requires holding the breath for 20 seconds after standard step test exercise; indicates the difference between normal pulse rate while standing and the pulse rate two minutes after exercise.

medial collaterals

The major binding ligaments on the sides of the knee joint and those criss-crossing from front to back within the joint; restrict sideward movement of the leg at the knee joint; the ligaments most often injured.

meditation

A method of relaxation; requires concentration, quiet, and repetition of prescribed thought patterns and words; transcendental meditation is the most widely known; Bhakti, Raji, and Kundalini yoga use meditation; can be used in combination with exercise or to prepare for exercise.

menarche

The beginning of menstruation.

mesomorph

A somatotype; a person with a body type characterized by muscular development and large prominent bones; often called an athletic body; other types are ectomorph and endomorph.

metabolic

Pertaining to metabolism.

metabolic fuel

A chemical or food used for energy production.

metabolism

The complex physical and chemical processes involved in the maintenance of life; the sum total of the chemical changes or reactions occurring in the body.

metabolite

Any substance produced by a metabolic reaction.

metacarpus

The part of the hand or foot that includes the five bones between the phalanges and the carpus.

metatarsus

The middle part of the foot in man, composed of the five bones between the toes and the tarsus; forms the instep.

micronutrients

Vitamins and minerals; necessary to the diet in small amounts.

midriff

The diaphragm; the middle, outer portion of the front of the human body, extending roughly from just below the breast to the waistline.

mileage

The distance a runner or any exerciser goes during an exercise session; e.g., marathon runners often run more than 100 miles a week during training; bicycle riders often ride more than 300 miles per week.

military press

A weight-lifting exercise in which the barbell is pressed upward from the chest until the arms are fully extended over the head. The weight is then lowered to the starting position; strengthens the deltoid and tricep muscles.

minerals

Inorganic compounds, some of which are nutrients (i.e., vital to proper bodily function); important nutrient minerals are calcium, phosphorus, potassium, sodium, iron, and iodine.

mitochondria

Slipper-shaped cell bodies that are the seat of the aerobic manufacture of ATP energy; muscle cells are rich in mitochondria; referred to as the "powerhouses" of the cell; the singular is mitochondrion.

motoneuron

A nerve cell that, when stimulated, causes muscular contraction; also called motor neuron or motor nerve.

motor cortex

An area of the brain that contains specialized neurons that cause motor movement when stimulated.

motor fitness

A group of traits, including muscular endurance, agility, speed, running endurance, and others that are used to determine levels of fitness.

motor nerve

See *motoneuron*.

Mr. America

An annual contest for bodybuilders; contestants are judged on several counts; body symmetry (the overall development of the body's musculature) is the goal and the primary determinant in judging and selecting winners; contests are judged in lightweight, middleweight, and heavyweight classes; points are accumulated in three phases—prejudging, mandatory posing, and free posing; Mr. Universe and Mr. Olympia are the other major bodybuilding titles in the world competition; hundreds of other bodybuilding contests are held annually; women bodybuilders also compete for similar titles.

Mr. Olympia

See *Mr. America*.

Mr. Universe

See *Mr. America*.

muscle

A tissue composed of fibers capable of contracting and relaxing to effect bodily movement; principal types are striated (e.g., the bicep), smooth (e.g., the intestines), and the cardiac, or heart muscle; movement is not possible without muscular activity; there are more than 600 muscles in the body.

muscle-bound

A term applied to people with large musculature; until the 1940s it was generally thought that excessive weight training brought about a condition of limited flexibility or muscle boundness; the condition was considered to have an adverse effect on athletic performance. The theory is now discredited, as weight trainers have been shown to have greater flexibility than many normally developed people.

muscle cell

The basic contractile unit at work in all activities involving flexing, extending, bending, and so on; also called muscle fiber; muscle fibers may be fast to contract or slow to contract (see *fast-twitch fibers* and *slow-twitch fibers*).

muscle cramps

Painful contractions of the muscle fibers; can last for a few seconds or several hours; usually occur during exercise; may be caused by low levels of potassium and salt.

muscle fiber

An elongated, contractile cell, highly striated.

muscle imbalance

A condition in which opposing muscles are not of equal strength; when one muscle moves in one direction another muscle moves in the opposite direction; when one muscle is stronger than the other it can overpower the weaker one and cause damage to fibers and tendons.

muscle pull

An acute tear of muscle fibers; results in sudden localized pain; can be caused by insufficient warm-up, overtraining, muscle imbalance, or poor flexibility.

muscle spasm

See *cramp.*

muscle spindle

A proprioceptor located in a muscle fiber (see *proprioceptor*).

muscular endurance

The ability of a muscle or muscle group to perform repeated contractions against a light load for an extended period of time; this work may be performed either by sustained muscular contractions (isometric) or by continuing to raise and lower a submaximal load (isotonic) as in weight training; one of the three primary elements of physical fitness, along with muscular strength and circulatory-respiratory endurance.

muscular power

The ability to release maximum muscular force in the shortest time, e.g., in the standing broad jump or a vertical leap.

muscular strength

Strength of muscles as determined by a single maximum muscle contraction measured with calibrated instruments such as dynamometers or tensiometers (see *dynamometer* and *tensiometer*).

muscular tension

The feeling of tightness in a muscle that has been exercised; also describes the state of the muscle during contraction.

musculature

The system of muscles throughout the body.

myelin sheath

A structure composed mainly of lipid (fat) and protein that surrounds some nerve fibers (axons).

myocardium

The muscle tissue of the heart.

myocardium blood supply

The blood supply to the heart, delivered through a special set of arteries called the coronary arteries.

myofibril

That part of a muscle fiber containing two protein filaments, myosin and actin.

myology

The study of muscles.

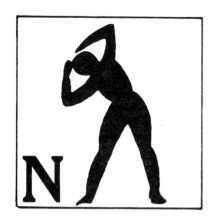

nausea

A feeling of the need to vomit; usually caused by a strong stomach disturbance; can result from overexertion.

Nautilus

The trademark name of exercise machines invented by Arthur Jones that provide progressive resistance exercise; designed around a system of cams, this equipment is easier to use than conventional weight training equipment (barbells) because each movement is guided by the machine; provides a controlled workout for the beginner or the experienced weight lifter; expensive equipment, therefore not suitable for home use.

navicular

A comma-shaped bone of the wrist; the concave bone in front of the anklebone on the instep of the foot.

negative work

In weight lifting, lowering the weight is considered negative work; the muscles are lengthened; e.g., in lowering the bar from a curl.

nerve

A cord-like structure that conveys impulses from one part of the body to another; any of the bundles of fibers connecting the central nervous system and the organs or parts of the body; transmits both sensory stimuli and motor impulses from one part of the body to another; the source of feeling, energy, or dynamic action.

nerve cell

Any of the cells of nerve tissue consisting of a nucleated portion and cytoplasmic extensions, the cell body, the dendrites, and axons; also called a neuron.

nerve center

A group of nerve cells that perform a specific function.

nerve fiber

A threadlike part of the nerve; an axon or dendrite, each of which is capable of conducting nervous impulses.

nerve impulse

An electrical disturbance at the point of stimulation of a nerve that is transmitted along the entire length of the axon.

nervous system

The system of nerves and nerve centers, including the central (voluntary) nervous system and the autonomic (involuntary) nervous system; coordinates and regulates internal bodily functions and the body's responses to outside stimuli; connects the brain, spinal cord, nerves, and receptor organs.

neural

Pertaining to the nerves.

neuromuscular

Refers to both the nervous and muscular systems; the systems must work in concert for general movement and especially for good sports performance.

neuron

A conducting cell of the nervous system consisting of a cell body (with its nucleus and cytoplasm), dendrites, and an axon.

New York City Marathon

The largest marathon in the U.S. with more than 17,000 runners; the course goes through the five boroughs of New York City (see *marathon*).

niacin

A vitamin that works with thiamin and riboflavin in energy-producing reactions in cells; found in liver, poultry, meat, tuna, whole grain and enriched cereals, bread, nuts, dried beans, and peas.

norepinephrine

See *adrenaline.*

nutrient

Something that nourishes, especially a nourishing ingredient in a food.

nutriment

Anything that nourishes; food; anything that aids growth or development.

nutrition

The process of nourishing or being nourished; especially, the interrelated steps by which a living organism assimilates food and uses it for growth and replacement of tissues; the study of food, vitamin, and mineral requirements.

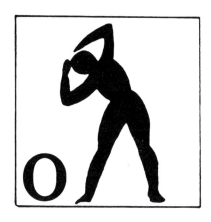

obese

Extremely fat; more than 25% over ideal weight (see *ideal weight*).

Ohio State University Step Test

A progressive step test, continued until the heart rate reaches 150 beats per minute; similar to the Harvard step test (see *Harvard step test*).

Olympic lifting

A series of two-barbell lifts performed in national and international competitions; lifts are the snatch and the clean and jerk; the snatch is performed by picking the weight up from the floor and pressing it over the head in one continuous motion while either splitting or bending the legs; the clean and jerk is performed by bringing the weight from the floor to shoulder height in one movement, either splitting or bending the legs and then pressing up until the arms are fully extended over the head; contestants are divided into 10 weight classes; the person lifting the most total weight in the two lifts wins the competition; in higher weight classifications, records total more than 900 pounds.

omnivorous

Feeding on both animal and vegetable substances.

organic

Used to describe food products that are grown without the use of artificial or chemical fertilizers; the proponents of organic foods say such foods have more nutritional value than nonorganic foods; products that are organically grown are also called "natural" or "health" foods; they are carried in specialty stores and are usually priced higher than non-organic food items.

orthopedics
The surgical or manipulative treatment of disorders of the skeletal system and other motor organs.

orthopedist
A physician who specializes in orthopedics; often called upon to assist athletes with joint problems.

orthotics
Rigid or flexible inserts in shoes that provide support and stabilization; made from a plaster mold of the foot; used to treat knee, back, hip, and ankle conditions; usually prescribed by podiatrists and orthopedists.

Osler, William
First professor of medicine at Johns Hopkins University; once said, "Patients should have rest, food, fresh air, and exercise—the quadrangle of health."

ossification
The natural process of bone formation; the abnormal hardening or calcification of soft tissue into a bonelike material as in calcium deposits in and around joints; a mass or deposit of such material.

osteoarthritis
A condition that results from a thinning of the spinal disks and the growth of small, bony protuberances that press against the sciatic nerve (see *sciatic nerve*); a cause of back pain; degenerative arthritis usually concentrates in the larger joints.

osteoclasis
Surgical fracture of a bone performed to correct a deformity.

osteomalacia
Softening of the bones because of a deficiency of Vitamin D or of calcium and phosphorus.

osteomyelitis
Inflammation of the bone marrow.

osteopathy
A medical therapy that emphasizes manipulation of the joints as a technique for correcting physical abnormalities.

osteoporosis
The weakening of the bones as people age; often results in broken bones, especially in the legs and hips; research indicates the process may be slowed or prevented with exercise.

overdevelop
To develop to excess; usually used in reference to muscular development; bodybuilding champions and bodybuilders are thought by some to be overdeveloped.

overexert
To exert too much; to exhaust; can result in injury or fatigue.

overhand grip
The palms-in method of holding a barbell, dumbbell, or chinning bar.

overload
To exercise a muscle or muscle group against resistance greater than that which is normally encountered; to add more weight or resistance as strength increases, e.g., when it becomes easy to lift 50 pounds, 10 more pounds can be added for the exercise; resistance can be maximal or near-maximal; overload is what produces muscle growth or hypertrophy; the heart muscle can also be overloaded and strengthened through aerobic exercise (see *training effects*).

overtraining
A condition that develops when an exerciser trains too hard for too many days; symptoms include dull aches in the joints and muscles during workouts, continued pain after workouts, heavy-leggedness, headaches, loss of appetite, depression, and nervousness; rest is the primary treatment.

overweight

Weighing more than is normal or necessary, anywhere from 5-15% above ideal weight (see *ideal weight*).

oxidize

To combine with oxygen.

oxidizer

Any substance that oxidizes or induces another substance to oxidize.

oxygen

Colorless, odorless, tasteless element essential for respiration; combines with most other elements; constitutes 21% of the atmosphere.

oxygen consumption

The intake and utilization of oxygen by the body; measured by maximum oxygen uptake (VO_2max) (see *maximum oxygen uptake*).

oxygen debt

The amount of oxygen consumed during recovery from exercise above that ordinarily consumed at rest in the same time period. Blood flow through the muscle is impaired while the muscle is in tension or contracted. Much of the energy cost of its contraction, if it is held very long, causes oxygen debt in the muscle that must be repaid in the form of oxygen flow after the muscle has relaxed; accompanying the increased oxygen consumption are increases in the rate and depth of breathing, heart rate, cardiac output, and body temperature; oxygen debt includes two components: lactacid, which is related to removal of lactic acid from the muscles and blood, and alactacid, which provides the necessary oxygen for the restoration of phosphagens (ATP and PC).

oxygen transport system

The cardio-respiratory system, which controls oxygen intake and delivery to the muscles; components include oxygen intake, stroke volume, and heart rate; most important during endurance exercise.

oxyhemoglobin

A bright-red chemical complex of hemoglobin and oxygen; transports oxygen from the lungs to the tissues through the blood.

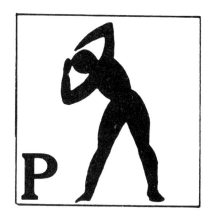

pacemaker
A mass of specialized muscle fibers of the heart that regulate the heartbeat; artificial pacemakers are electrical devices for steadying or stimulating the action of the heart.

palpitate
Refers to the quivering or fluttering of the heart; to beat more quickly than usual; throb.

parallel bars
Two bars, 16″ apart and 5′3″ off the floor used for a variety of gymnastic exercises.

pasta
A paste in processed or dough form, e.g., spaghetti; a source of carbohydrates that is often consumed in quantity by runners the night before a long race such as a half marathon or a marathon (see *carbohydrate loading*).

patella
A flat, triangular bone located at the front of the knee joint; also called kneecap.

P.B.
See *personal best.*

peaking
The period from several weeks to a few days before a competi-

tion when training time is reduced but the intensity of the exercise is increased.

pecs
Slang term used by bodybuilders and other athletes for the pectoral muscles of the chest.

pectoral
Pertaining to the breast or chest; usually used in reference to large chest muscles; also called pecs.

pedometer
A device for measuring the distance traveled on foot; attaches to the waist and adjusted for stride length; useful for runners and other exercisers.

peds
Low-cut athletic socks that cover the foot but do not come over the ankle; favored by runners because they are cool and lightweight.

pelvic tilt
An exercise; performed from the supine position with knees flexed at 45° and feet flat on the floor; the abdomen is pulled in and the pelvis is tilted upward with the weight supported by the shoulders until the lower spine is off the floor; strengthens the lumbar region of the lower back.

pelvis
Basin-shaped skeletal structure; composed of the bones on the sides, the pubis in front, and the sacrum and coccyx behind; rests on the lower limbs and supports the spinal column.

pep
Energy; high spirits; vigor.

pepsin
A digestive enzyme found in gastric juice that catalyzes the breakdown of protein to peptide.

peptide
Any of the natural or synthetic compounds containing two or more amino acids.

pericardium
The membranous sac enclosing the heart.

perimysium
The connective tissue that surrounds a muscle bundle (fasciculus).

perineum
The portion of the body in the pelvis occupied by urogenital passages and the rectum, bounded in front by the pubic arch, in the back by the coccyx, and laterally by part of the hip bone.

perineurium
A sheath of connective tissue enclosing a bundle of nerves.

peristalsis
The involuntary muscular waves of the intestine that move its contents along.

personal best (P.B.)
A personal record for an athletic endeavor; e.g., an individual's time for running a 10K race or the number of pounds lifted in a weight training exercise; usually of importance only to the individual.

personal record (P.R.)
See *personal best.*

Pheidippides
Famous Greek messenger (see *marathon* and *marathon stone*).

phosphagens
Compounds that release energy when broken down; ATP and PC are phosphagens.

phosphatide
Any of a group of lipid (fat) compounds, such as lecithin and

cephalin, composed mainly of glycerol and phosphoric acid, and found in great abundance with stored fats in plant and animal tissues.

phys ed

See *physical education.*

physiatrist

A physician (M.D.) specializing in the rehabilitation of the physically disabled, including postoperative patients; responsibilities include prescription of exercise for such patients.

physical

Pertaining to the body, as distinguished from the mind or spirit; a complete medical examination.

physical culture

A study and practice of activities thought to contribute to health, nutrition, and well-being; popular in the late 1800s and early 1900s; promoted natural methods, personal care, and exercise; Bernarr MacFadden was its best-known proponent.

Physical Culture

A magazine founded by physical culturist Bernarr MacFadden in 1898, one of the first publications devoted exclusively to health and fitness and emphasizing exercise and nutrition.

physical education

The generic name given to a variety of programs required of students in most high schools and colleges; commonly called phys ed and aimed at those not actively participating in formal athletics; activities range from sports such as volleyball, tumbling, and basketball to calisthenics and track and field; usually includes classroom lectures on subjects relating to health and fitness; has often been controversial because of inclusion of materials about sex and reproduction; such courses originated before the Civil War and included tests that measured aspects of physical fitness; after World War I, activities broadened to include play, games, and sports with an emphasis on motor effectiveness.

physical fitness

See *fitness*.

Physical Fitness Research Digest

A publication of the President's Council on Physical Fitness and Sports that ceased publication in 1979; reported on subjects relating to health, fitness, and well-being; each issue devoted to a specific area of interest, e.g., development of muscular strength and endurance, joint and body range of movement, and the totality of man.

physical therapist

A practitioner of therapy that is designed to develop physiological processes such as strength, flexibility, endurance; important in the area of rehabilitation from exercise and sports injuries.

physiology

The biological science of essential life processes, activities, and functions.

physique

The body considered with reference to its proportions, muscular development, and appearance.

physique contests

Public exhibitions of muscular development with participation by men and women; contests conducted in all areas of the world (see *Mr. America*).

pinch test

A test for body fat; use of the forefinger and the thumb to pinch the fat away from the muscle in the area behind the bicep, at the waist, and on the front of the thigh; gives approximate determination of the amount of fat and amount of lean body mass (see *skinfold caliper*).

pit stop

The euphemism for stopping to go to the bathroom during an athletic event; used primarily by runners.

pituitary gland

A small, oval endocrine gland attached to the base of a vertebrate's brain, whose secretions control the other endocrine glands and influence growth, metabolism, and maturity.

plantar fasciitis

A tear and inflammation of the tissues called fasciae, which protect nerves and muscles; a common athletic injury caused by a slight tear of the fascia that covers the muscles on the bottom of the feet; usually causes pain under the heel bone; can be treated with rest or by wearing special shoes that offer additional support for the arch.

plasma

The clear, yellowish liquid portion of the blood, lymph, or intramuscular fluid in which cells are suspended.

platelets

One of the three solid elements of blood that are visible under an ordinary microscope; others are red cells and white cells; promote clotting.

plates

The term used to describe the weights that are placed on barbells and dumbbells; vary in weight from ½ pound to 100 pounds; also called barbell plates (see *barbells*).

pleura

Either of two membranous sacs which line each side of the thoracic cavity and envelop the lung, reducing the friction of respiratory movements to a minimum.

plexus

A structure in the form of a network, especially of nerves, blood vessels, or lymphatics found in several parts of the body including the abdomen, the thorax, and the cervix (see *solar plexus*).

plump

Well-rounded and full in form; chubby.

podiatrist

A medical doctor who studies and treats foot ailments; also called a chiropodist.

pommel horse

A piece of equipment used in gymnastics; a raised padded "horse" with two handles; provides a platform that allows the gymnast to make swings, circles, and other moves.

portal vein

A vein that conducts blood from the digestive organs, spleen, pancreas, and gall bladder to the liver.

positive addiction

The term applied to compulsive exercisers because, unlike drug or alcohol addiction, exercise is beneficial.

positive work

In weight lifting, raising the weight is considered positive work; the muscles are shortened.

posture

The position or attitude of the body; the muscles of the stomach and back are important to good posture.

power

Work per unit of time; e.g., if 1 kilogram is raised 1 meter in 1 second, power is expressed as 1 kilogram-meter per second; a measure of strength.

power bench

Used primarily for performing the bench press exercise (see *bench*).

power clean

A weight-lifting exercise in which the barbell is brought up from floor to the chest in one continuous movement; strengthens the quadriceps.

power rack

A device that aids in the performance of isometric exercises; the exerciser uses a barbell that fits inside two vertical poles that guide the bar; the vertical poles have holes at intervals where metal pins can be inserted, limiting the movement of the barbell; e.g., for the military press the pins are inserted at the arms-extended position over the head—the exerciser presses the barbell against the pins and holds it in place for the required length of time; most weight-lifting movements can be performed to achieve isometric results (see *isometrics*).

P.R.
See *personal best.*

PRE
See *progressive resistance exercise.*

preacher bench
A small bench designed to isolate the biceps muscles while performing the biceps curl; the upper part of the arm is placed on the bench for the exercise; so called because it resembles a preacher's podium.

President's Council on Physical Fitness and Sports
An organization established by President Dwight D. Eisenhower to inform the public about the issues of physical fitness and the need for health and exercise; established because of concern for the fitness of America's youth following comparison tests with European children conducted in the 1950s; originally called President's Council on Youth Fitness.

press behind neck
A weight-lifting exercise in which the barbell is pressed upward from the back of the neck until the arms are fully extended over the head; the weight is then lowered to the starting position; strengthens the deltoid and triceps muscles (see *military press*).

pressure
The application of continuous force by one body upon another; compression; force applied over a surface; measured as force per unit of area.

prime mover
The contracting muscle in any movement; e.g., in flexing the

elbow, the biceps muscle contracts (prime mover) and the triceps muscle (antagonist) relaxes (see *antagonist*).

procrastinate

To put off doing something until later; procrastination is used extensively by exercisers to postpone workouts.

progress

Movement toward a goal; development.

progressive resistance exercise (PRE)

The gradual increase in the amount of resistance against which a given muscle or muscle group must work as the strength of the muscle improves; necessary in order to maintain a high level of tension; overloading of a muscle or muscle group (see *overload*).

pronate

To turn the palm or inner surface of the hand or leg downward or backward.

pronated feet

A condition in which the feet roll inward excessively; caused by weak ankles; sometimes called flat feet, although the feet are not really flat; orthotics are used for treatment (see *orthotics*).

pronator

The forearm or leg muscle that effects pronation (see *pronate*).

proportion

A relationship between things or parts of things with respect to comparative magnitude, quantity, or degree; harmonious relation, balance, symmetry; important in bodybuilding and muscular development.

proprioceptors

Sense organs that are found in muscle joints and tendons and that give information concerning movement and body position (kinethesis) to the central nervous system; muscle spindles are proprioceptors.

prostatitis

A swelling of the prostate gland that causes painful urination; a potential side effect of the carbohydrate-loading phase of training for long-distance running events.

protein

Any of a group of complex organic compounds of high molecular weight that contain amino acids as their basic structural units; occurs in all living matter; essential for growth and repair of tissue; one of the three macronutrients with carbohydrates and fats; ingesting one gram of protein per kilo (2.2 lbs.) of body weight per day is considered adequate for normal growth.

protoplasm

A complex, jellylike substance that constitutes plant and animal cells; all body tissue is composed of this substance.

psychomotor

Pertaining to muscular activity associated with the mental processes.

pulldown

An exercise performed with a machine with a bar and a cable that is attached to a weight; in the sitting or standing position, the exerciser pulls the bar down behind the neck or in front of the body; strengthens the latissimus dorsi muscles; also called lat pulldown.

pull-up

See *chin-up*.

pulse rate

The number of times the heart beats per minute; roughly the same as the heart rate (see *resting heart rate*).

push-up

An exercise performed lying face down; with weight on hands and toes, the body is raised from the floor until arms are fully extended; the back is flat; strengthens arm, shoulder, and abdominal muscles.

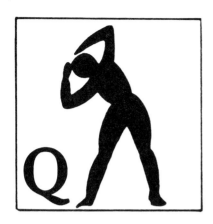

quadriceps femoris
The muscle that forms the main bulk of the front of the thigh.

quads
A slang term used by bodybuilders and other athletes for the quadriceps muscles in the front of the upper thigh.

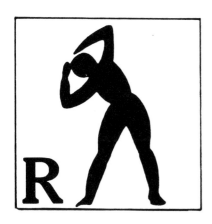

race walker

A person who walks swiftly for exercise or in competition; rules require that one foot must be in contact with the ground at all times; no running is allowed; also called heel and toe because the walker first places the heel on the ground, then rolls to the toe.

racing flats

A type of ultra light, flexible jogging shoe that is designed for racing only; not as durable as the basic jogging shoe.

racquetball

A racquet game played in an enclosed, four-walled court by two or four players; the ball is hollow and pressurized and the racquets can be no more than 27″ long; the ball may hit any or all walls; points are scored when the ball bounces more than once on the floor; good exercise, but only average for cardiovascular fitness.

radius

A long, prismatic, slightly curved bone; the shorter and thicker of the two forearm bones.

range of motion

The term applied to the ability to move the limbs freely around the joints; flexibility.

RDAs

See *Recommended Dietary Allowances*.

reaction time

The time necessary to respond to a stimulus; commonly tested by having a subject press or release a button as quickly as possible after seeing a flashing light; used to test reflexes; a fit person has better reaction time than an unfit person, regardless of age.

receptor

A nerve ending specialized to sense or to receive stimuli.

Recommended Dietary Allowances (RDAs)

The U.S. government's guidelines for the maintenance of good nutrition; the RDAs include suggested levels of calories, protein, calcium, phosphorus, iron, Vitamin A, thiamin, riboflavin, niacin, and ascorbic acid.

recovery heart rate

The heart rate that is reached 5 to 15 minutes after vigorous exercise; should be within 20 beats of pre-exercise levels or approximately 100 beats per minute within that time period; the faster the recovery rate the more fit the cardiovascular system.

recovery time

The period necessary for the exerciser to regenerate the body's fuel, muscles, and reserves; physiologists are not in agreement, but most suggest at least 24 hours for recovery after strenuous exercise.

recreational sports

Activities such as golf, bowling, and softball that provide exercise but do relatively little for cardiovascular fitness.

rectus

Any of the various straight muscles, as of the abdomen, eye, neck, and thigh.

rectus abdominus

See *abdominal muscles.*

rectus femoris

The muscle that occupies the central portion of the quadriceps femoris, the four-part muscle forming the main bulk of the front of the thigh.

red blood cells

The cells in the blood that contain hemoglobin and are responsible for carrying oxygen (see *white blood cells*).

reduce

To lose weight through dieting and/or exercise.

reference man

The term used to describe the average American man; dimensions are: height 5'9", weight 162 lbs., chest 39 inches, waist 32 inches, hips 38 inches.

reference woman

The term used to describe the average American woman; height 5'4", weight 135 lbs., chest 35 inches, waist 29 inches.

reflex

An automatic response induced by stimulation of a receptor or nerve ending (see *reaction time*).

regenerate

Restore, refresh, renew.

relax

To become lax or loose; to relieve tension or stress; exercise provides relaxation for many people.

relief interval

In an interval training program, the time between bouts of work; also the time between sets of lifts during weight training (see *interval training*).

repetition

The number of times an exercise is performed; often used to describe the movements in weight training; in weight training the same exercise, e.g., a military press, may be performed 8 to 15 times, or repetitions; a specified number of repetitions make a set of exercises; there are usually three sets of a series of exercises in a complete workout.

repetition maximum (RM)

The maximum number of times a given weight can be lifted through the full range of a given movement; e.g., a 10-repetition maximum exercise is designated as 10-RM, which indicates that a particular weight can be lifted just 10 times through the full range of motion of the involved joints before the muscles are fatigued; first formulated by Thomas L. DeLorme, a pioneer in the use of resistance exercise in physical rehabilitation medicine.

repetition running

Similar to interval training but with longer runs and longer rests between runs (see *interval training*).

reps

See *repetition*.

resistance

The amount of weight or pressure involved in any exercise; e.g., a barbell with 20 pounds has greater resistance than a 10-pound dumbbell.

respiration

Breathing; the act of inhaling and exhaling; ventilation of the lungs and respiratory system.

resting heart rate

The rate at which the heart beats when movement is minimal; the average resting heart rate for men is 60 to 80 beats per minute and for women the rate is 70 to 90; a fit person's rate may be 60 per minute or less; the resting heart rate will drop after a few weeks of aerobic exercise; a low resting heart rate is a sign of good physical fitness.

reverse curl

A barbell or dumbbell exercise; the weight is held with the palms facing down; the weight is then raised from the arms-extended position until it touches the chest; strengthens the biceps and forearms; (see *curl*).

reverse wrist curl

See *reverse curl* and *wrist curl*.

reversibility
The fact that a lifetime of exercise does not insure against the loss of condition if exercise is stopped; losses occur in as little as a few weeks.

rheumatoid arthritis
A disease that results in the gradual deterioration of the joints; can lead to permanent stiffness and debility; more likely to affect younger people and women than osteoarthritis (see *osteoarthritis*).

riboflavin
A vitamin necessary for the release of energy to cells from carbohydrates, proteins, and fats; found in liver, milk, meat, dark green vegetables, whole grain and enriched cereals, bread, and mushrooms.

RICE
An acronym for rest, ice, compression, and elevation, the recommended immediate treatment for most sports injuries; rest is necessary because continued exercise could cause further injury; ice decreases bleeding from injured blood vessels; compression (or pressure) limits swelling; elevation of the injured part to a position above the level of the heart uses gravity to help drain excess fluid from the affected area.

rickets
A deficiency disease characterized by defective bone growth resulting from a lack of Vitamin D and from insufficient exposure to sunlight; occurs chiefly in children.

rings
Used in gymnastics; two rings suspended 8′ 2″ from the floor; used for a variety of gymnastic exercises.

ripped
A term used by bodybuilders to indicate a positive physical condition that is characterized by low body fat and extreme muscular development; subcutaneous fat is virtually eliminated and veins and blood vessels are clearly visible, hence the ripped condition.

Ripper

The trademark name of one of a variety of products in the shape of a small pocket that are attached to the laces of a shoe; designed to carry the keys and money of a person engaged in an athletic event; especially useful for runners.

RM

See *repetition maximum.*

robust

Full of health and strength; vigorous; fit.

Rolfing

A method of massage to realign the body that applies intensive pressure to the muscles; can be painful.

roller machine

A passive exercise aid that consists of a barrel-shaped base with wooden rollers; the exerciser sits on the rollers as the drum is turned by a motor; not useful for fitness purposes.

rope skipping

A method of aerobic exercise; traditional rope jumping that is adapted for cardiovascular fitness establishing jumping routines that are of sufficient duration (10-20 minutes) to stimulate the heart; recommended for people who have difficulty running because of knee problems; used extensively by boxers for the development of cardiovascular fitness and endurance.

roughage

The relatively coarse, indigestible parts of certain foods such as vegetables and unprocessed grains that contain cellulose and stimulate intestinal movement; fiber is also considered roughage (see *fiber*).

rowing

A method of aerobic exercise; may be done in a boat called a scull or with a rowing machine; strengthens the upper body and the arms (see *rowing machine*).

rowing machine

A device designed to imitate the motions of rowing; models

with stationary and sliding seats are available; may have adjustable resistance; usually portable and easily stored.

Royal Canadian Air Force Plans for Physical Fitness

The 5BX and XBX programs of progressive calisthenic exercises developed by the RCAF in 1962; extremely popular; designed to increase muscle tone, not to develop cardiovascular fitness.

rubdown

An energetic massage of the body; excellent for relaxing the muscles after exercise.

run

To move on foot at a pace faster than the walk and in such a manner that both feet leave the ground during each stride.

Run For Your Life

A program initiated by Dr. Gabe Mirkin in Baltimore, Maryland in 1963; now sponsored by the Road Runners Club of America, the program is for people of all ages and abilities who run for fun and fitness.

runner's bra

A bra especially constructed for female runners to prevent tearing of delicate breast tissue; has additional support and minimizes bounce; lined to prevent skin irritation.

runner's high

A euphoric condition that effects some runners after about 30 minutes of running; in some cases it may be a psychological condition and in others it may be caused by the release of chemicals inside the body and the brain (see *beta-endorphin*).

runner's knee

A condition caused by excessive pronation (flat feet); pronation causes more than normal twisting of the knee, which causes the kneecap to rub against the long bone of the thigh; results in pain behind the knee; can be treated with orthotics or rest (see *orthotics*).

runner's nipple

An irritation that results from the friction of a shirt against the nipples; can be treated by rubbing petroleum jelly on nipples prior to running.

runner's toe

Black toenails; results from continuous rubbing of the toes on the shoes; usually painless, but can result in losing the toenail; also called Morton's syndrome.

running shoes

Any of a wide variety of lightweight, well-cushioned shoes designed specifically for long-distance running; soles are of various designs and uppers are nylon, leather, or suede; the special cushioning provides support and lessens the impact of the foot on the ground surface during exercise.

running shorts

Nylon or cotton shorts, often with an inner pant liner; have elastic or tie waistband; usually have high-cut sides for ease of movement.

rupture

A tear of bodily tissue; especially in the groin area.

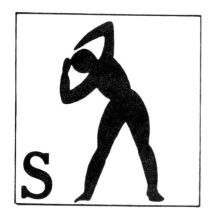

saccharin

A white, chemically formulated crystalline powder, having a taste about 500 times sweeter than cane sugar; used as a calorie-free sweetener; found to cause cancer in laboratory animals.

sacrum

A triangular bone consisting of five fused vertebrae that forms the posterior section of the pelvis.

sag

To diminish in firmness or strength, as in sagging muscles.

saliva

The watery, tasteless liquid mixture of salivary and oral mucous gland secretions that lubricate chewed food; moistens the oral walls and contains the enzyme ptyalin, which functions in the predigestion of starches.

sallow

Of a sickly, yellowish hue or complexion.

salt

Sodium chloride; absolutely necessary for many bodily functions; some salt can be lost in sweat during vigorous exercise or manual labor; salt loss can be replaced by eating a balanced diet; generally no additional salt in the form of tablets is necessary either before or after exercise; too much salt can be a cause of high blood pressure.

salt tablets

Sodium chloride in tablet form; formerly recommended for the replacement of salt loss in the form of sweat during exercise; no longer suggested for this purpose because too much salt in the system can cause high blood pressure or clots in the bloodstream.

salve

An ointment for soothing wounds or sores and protecting against bacterial infection.

sarcolemma

The cell membrane of a muscle fiber.

sarcomere

The smallest functional unit of muscle.

sarcoplasm

The protoplasm of muscle cells (see *protoplasm*).

sarcous

Pertaining to flesh or muscle.

sartorius

The flat, narrow thigh muscle, the longest muscle of the human anatomy, crossing the front of the thigh obliquely from the hip to the inner side of the tibia (shin).

sauna

A dry steam treatment originated in Finland; heat is usually produced by water poured on hot rocks; temperatures reach 175^0 or more; short exposures are recommended; a room for taking this type of treatment.

sauna belts

Waist cinchers made of rubber or plastic that are designed to induce sweat during exercise; not useful for fitness purposes; can be dangerous because they do not allow for the normal evaporation of sweat.

scapula

Either of two large flat triangular bones forming the back part of the shoulder; the shoulder blade.

scar tissue

A dense, often hard layer of connective tissue formed over a wound or cut.

Schneider Test

A measurement of the reclining pulse rate, the pulse rate increase on standing, the standing pulse rate, the pulse rate immediately after a standard chair-stepping exercise, the return of the pulse rate to normal after exercise, and the increase in systolic blood pressure from reclining to standing.

sciatica

Hip pain that radiates from the hip to the back of the thigh and leg; neuralgia of the sciatic nerve; may be caused by an unstable lower spine, a ruptured spinal disk, or excessive exercise.

sciatic nerve

A sensory and motor nerve originating in the lower spinal column and running down through the pelvis and upper leg; can be injured or pinched causing sciatica (see *sciatica*).

scissors kick

A swimming kick used chiefly with the side stroke in which one leg is swung forward, the other bent back at the knee, and then both are straightened and snapped together.

sclerosis

A thickening or hardening of a body part such as an artery or the spinal cord, especially from tissue overgrowth or disease.

scoliosis

Abnormal curvature of the spine.

Scott and French Test

A flexibility test that measures trunk-hip range of movement.

second wind

A phenomenon usually described as a sudden transition from an ill-defined feeling of fatigue during the early or middle portions of a prolonged period of exercise to a more comfortable, less stressful feeling later in the exercise period; implies easier breathing, but may also include relief from muscular fatigue; may be the result of adjustments in the body's ventilation process, removal of lactic acid accumulated early in the exercise, and/or psychological factors; reactions are highly individualized.

sedentary

Characterized by much sitting and little exercise; a potentially dangerous state that may lead to overweight and heart disease.

self-discipline

Training and control of oneself and one's conduct, usually for personal improvement; a necessary ingredient in training and fitness programs.

sensorimotor

Pertaining to the functions of the sensing and motor activities.

set

In an interval training program, a group of work and relief intervals; in weight training, the number of repetitions performed consecutively without resting (see *interval training* and *repetition*).

shiatsu

A method of massage or muscle relaxation that utilizes pressure "points" of the thumbs, fingers, hands, knuckles, and elbows.

shin

The front part of the leg below the knee and above the ankle; the tibia.

shin splints

Microscopic tears of the leg muscles in the area of the ankle; often suffered by runners because of an imbalance between the calf muscles on the back of the leg and the smaller, weaker muscles on the front of the lower leg; can be very painful; require rest and strengthening of the shin muscles by exercises such as walking up stairs.

Shoe Goo

The trademark name of a substance that can be applied to the rubber soles of athletic shoes to repair worn spots or reinforce areas that receive excessive wear.

Shorter, Frank

The winner of the marathon in the Olympics in 1972; credited with generating the interest in long-distance running in America.

shoulder

The part of the body between the neck and the upper arm.

shoulder blade

See *scapula.*

shoulder girdle

The area of the upper body stabilized by the muscles of the chest.

shoulder shrug

An exercise performed with a barbell in the arms-extended position in front of the body; the shoulders are shrugged, pulling the weight up; strengthens the trapezius muscles; sometimes called the shrug.

shrug

See *shoulder shrug.*

SI

See *strength index.*

sidestroke

A swimming stroke in which a person swims on one side and thrusts the arms forward alternately while performing a scissors kick (see *scissors kick*).

sinew

A tendon.

singlet

A nylon or cotton running shirt that has no sleeves; designed for ease of arm movement.

sit-ups

See *bent-knee sit-ups.*

skating

A method of exercise that can be performed on roller or ice skates.

skeletal muscle

The muscles of the body that are visible and can be developed through physical exercise.

skeleton

The internal vertebrate structure composed of bone and cartilage that protects and supports the soft organs, tissues, and other parts of the body.

skin

The 7-layer membranous tissue forming the external covering of the body; epidermis.

skinfold

A pinch of skin and subcutaneous fat from which total body fat may be estimated; measured with skinfold calipers or by a pinch test with the fingers (see *pinch test*).

skinfold caliper

A device much like a pair of pliers, used to measure the fat content of the body; measures thickness of a fold of skin pulled away from the muscle; skin is pinched at the waist, frontal thigh, and clavicle; readings indicate the amount of body fat and are calibrated in millimeters.

skinfold measurements

The readings taken with a skinfold caliper; results are measured in millimeters (see *skinfold caliper*).

slender

Having little width in proportion to the height or length; slim.

slipped disk

Popular term for a condition that develops when the cartilage between the vertebrae cracks and pushes against a nerve, especially the sciatic nerve; not actually the slippage of a disk; a cause of severe back pain.

slow twitch fibers

Red muscle fibers that are considered slower acting; have low anaerobic capacity, and high aerobic capacity; suited for low-power output activities; more prevalent in athletes who participate in sports events like the marathon that require endurance (see *fast-twitch fibers*).

sluggish

Displaying little movement or activity; slow; inactive; lacking energy.

small intestine

The part of the intestine in which digestion is completed; consists of the duodenum, the jejunum, and the ileum.

smooth muscle

The unstriated, involuntary muscles of the internal organs (excluding the heart), as of the intestine, bladder, and blood vessels. These muscles are not subject to development.

snatch

One of the required lifts in Olympic weight lifting competition (see *Olympic lifting*).

solar plexus

The large network of sympathetic nerves and ganglia located in the peritoneal cavity behind the stomach and having branching tracts that supply nerves to the abdominal viscera.

somatic

Of or pertaining to the body, especially as distinguished from a bodily part, the mind, or the environment.

somatotype

One or more body types (see *ectomorph*, *endomorph* or *mesomorph*).

somatotyping

The practice or method of identifying body types—mesomorphic, ectomorphic, or endomorphic—using a standard formula.

somersault

An acrobatic stunt in which the body rolls in a complete circle, heels over head.

soreness

A feeling of light to moderate pain in the muscles; the natural reaction of muscles to the strain of exercise; apparently caused by the slight tearing of muscle tissue; usually disappears within 48 hours; can be treated with creams and ointments.

spa

An expensive private club that provides a variety of health-oriented activities for people who may be members or who visit for a specified period of time; services available usually include supervised exercises such as aerobics, swimming, and weight lifting; special diets are often enforced; sometimes referred to as "fat farms."

space foil

An ultra-thin sheet of silver foil like kitchen foil that traps body heat; used for warming runners and other athletes after performances; is both inexpensive and disposable.

spasm

A sudden, involuntary contraction of a muscle or group of muscles; often occurs during or after bouts of exercise.

spasmodic

Pertaining to the character of a spasm; a tightening.

specificity

Refers to the theory that exercise is specific to the muscles that are being exercised and the best exercise for an athletic event is the event itself; i.e., the transfer of the effects of one type of training to another form of training is only partial; e.g., improvements in conditioning on the treadmill do not correlate with improvements on the bicycle ergometer; having effects that are directly linked to the particulars of training; the nontransferability of training from one sport to another, e.g., trained long-distance runners are not necessarily equally trained for long-distance cycling.

speed

The rapidity with which successive movements of the same kind can be performed.

speed play

An exercise program involving alternating fast and slow running, especially over natural terrains; designed to give runners a break from the regular routine of long, slow distance training, which can be boring and fatiguing (see *fartlek*).

sphincter

A ringlike muscle that normally maintains constriction of a bodily passage or orifice and that relaxes as required by normal physiological functioning.

spinal column

The columnar assemblage or articulated vertebrae extending from the cranium to the coccyx or the end of the tail bone, encases the spinal cord, and forms the supporting axis of the body; the backbone; also called vertebral column.

spinal cord

The part of the central nervous system contained within the spinal column; continuous at its cranial end with the medulla oblongata

spinal disk

See *slipped disk.*

splanchnic ptosis

A term that describes the increase in pulse rate and systolic blood pressure from the sitting to the standing position or from lying to standing.

spleen

One of the largest lymphoid structures in the body; a visceral organ composed of a white pulp of lymphatic nodules and tissue and a red pulp of venous sinusoids in a framework of fibrous partitions lying on the left side below the diaphragm; functions as a blood filter and blood storage area.

split time

The period of time it takes to run part of a distance; e.g., the time for ¼ of a mile in a mile run is a split time; each piece of a race or a workout can be timed in this manner.

spondylitis

Inflammation of one or more of the vertebrae; may result from injury or disease; causes stiffness in joints between the vertebrae and can cause deformation; a cause of back pain.

sports medicine

An area of medicine that deals with the physiological, anatomical, psychological, and biochemical effects of exercise; often includes other areas of concern such as training methods, injury prevention, injury treatment and rehabilitation and nutrition.

spot reducing

The theory that diet or a specific exercise can reduce fat in a part or parts of the body that have excess fat; specific exercise is prescribed for those areas; e.g., side bends are suggested for reducing the fat around the waist; discredited by physiologists and nutritionists because fat is stored and eliminated equally throughout the body.

spotter

In weight training and gymnastics, a person who assists the weight lifter or gymnast by helping him or her perform the exercises correctly and safely.

sprint

Running short dashes as fast as possible.

sprint training

A type of conditioning designed to increase the capacity of the anaerobic system needed for short, high-power activities such as sprints; can also be used in bouts of interval training for improvement in speed for long-distance running (see *interval training*).

squash

A racquet game played in an enclosed court by two or four players; racquets have long thin handles and small (9") heads; the ball is hard rubber, 1.56 to 1.63 inches in diameter; the ball may hit any wall and points are scored when the ball isn't hit after the first bounce on the floor.

squat

See *deep-knee bend.*

squat rack

Two vertical supports on which a weight-lifting bar can be rested both before and after the squat exercise.

stance

The attitude or position of a standing person especially the position assumed by an athlete or sportsman in action.

standing broad jump

A test of leg strength and part of the overall estimate of a person's level of fitness; performed by standing with the feet on a starting line in a squatting position and then springing forward as far as possible.

standing press

See *military press.*

starch

A naturally abundant nutrient carbohydrate found chiefly in seeds, fruits, tubers, roots, and stem pith of plants, notably in corn, potatoes, wheat, and rice; varies widely in appearance according to source; packaged as a white, amorphous, tasteless powder.

stationary bicycle

An exercise machine, usually with one wheel, that has an adjustable tension control that allows the exerciser to increase resistance; excellent for improving leg strength and cardiovascular fitness.

steambath

A wet-heat treatment; steam is produced by hot water or a hot-water machine; a room for taking this type of treatment.

sternum

The long flat bone that supports most of the ribs; also called breastbone.

steroid

Any of numerous naturally occurring, fat-soluble organic compounds having a 17-carbon atom ring as a basis, and including the sterols and bile acids; many hormones, certain natural drugs such as digitalis compounds, and the precursors of certain vitamins are included in the steroid group; synthetic anabolic (tissue-building) products originally developed to reverse the negative nitrogen balance that occurs in surgical and trauma patients; these drugs tend to keep the body from losing its muscle mass during periods of rest; a derivative of the male sex hormone testosterone, which has masculinizing properties; used by strength athletes and others who desire to build muscle mass quickly; can be taken in pill form or through injection; has negative side effects, possibly including cancer and sterility; also called anabolic steroids.

stiff-legged dead lift

An exercise performed by bending at the waist and picking up a barbell or dumbbell from the floor, then standing and lifting it to the arms-extended position; the knees are kept locked during the movement; the weight is then lowered back to the floor; strengthens the quadriceps; also called dead lift.

stimulant

Anything that temporarily arouses or accelerates physiological or organic activity; caffeine is the most common of these agents.

stitch

A sudden, sharp pain in the upper abdomen that is a form of muscle cramp generally due to indigestion or to poor circulation in the chest muscles; usually occurs during prolonged, repetitive exercise; can often be relieved by slow, deep breathing or bending backward from the waist (see *cramp*).

stomach

The enlarged, sac-like portion of the alimentary canal; one of the principal organs of digestion; located in vertebrates between the esophagus and the small intestine.

stopwatch

A timepiece, either digital or with a sweep second hand, used for timing sports events; gives results in 1/100th of a second.

straight arm pullover

An exercise performed from the supine position but with the arms straight instead of bent; strengthens the shoulder and chest muscles (see *pullover*).

straight leg sit-up

A sit-up performed from the lying position with the legs fully extended; strengthens the abdominal muscles (see *bent-knee sit-up*).

straight trunk sit-up

A sit-up performed with the trunk kept straight throughout the movement; strengthens the abdominal muscles (see *bent-knee sit-up*).

strawberry

A red skin abrasion often occurring on the knee or elbow and caused by a fall on an exercise mat, floor or ground (see *mat burn*).

strength

The maximal pulling force of a muscle or muscle group; the state, quality, or property of being strong; physical power, muscularity; usually refers to muscular strength; the ability of a muscle or muscle group to lift an object in a single maximum contraction; along with muscular endurance and circulatory-respiratory endurance, one of the three primary elements of physical fitness.

Strength & Health

A magazine, first published in 1932 by Bob Hoffman, the founder of York Barbell Company, York, PA.; focuses on subjects related to bodybuilding, weight lifting, nutrition, and health; edited by John Grimek, a former Mr. America.

strength index (SI)

Gross strength score derived by dividing the SI by a norm for the individual's age, sex, and weight; tests include lung capacity, right and left grip strengths, back and leg lifts, pull-ups, and push-ups.

stress

The amount of pressure placed on an organism; can be physical or mental.

stress fracture

A hairline crack in the surface of a bone, most often in the feet and legs; very painful and difficult to diagnose; caused by excessive running or other types of training; usually heals by itself.

stretch

To lengthen, widen, or distend by pulling; to flex the muscles.

stretching exercises

Any of a number of types of exercise movements that are designed to lengthen, tone, and warm the muscles; usually used as warm-up movements for other types of exercise, including aerobic exercise, and for cooldown movements following strenuous exercise; can be formulated to provide a complete exercise routine; basic to aerobic dance and calisthenic exercises.

striated muscle

Skeletal, voluntary, and cardiac muscle distinguished from smooth muscle by visible bands of protein on the muscle.

stroke volume

The amount of blood pumped by the heart per heat; at rest, the volume is between 70 and 80 milliliters per beat or approximately 5 to 6 liters per minute; volume can be as high as 35 liters per minute in highly trained endurance athletes during maximal exercise.

subcutaneous fat

Fat deposits stored directly beneath the skin.

submaximal exercise

Exercise demanding less than the maximal oxygen consumption of the person performing the exercise; most exercise is conducted at the submaximal level.

sucrose

A crystalline disaccharide carbohydrate found in many plants, mainly sugar cane, sugar beet, and maple, and used widely as a sweetener, preservative, and in the manufacture of plastics and cellulose; also called cane sugar and saccharose.

sudoriferous

Producing or secreting sweat.

sugar

A sweet crystalline carbohydrate (see *sucrose*).

supine

A position: lying on the back with the face upward.

supple

Readily bent, pliant; moving and bending with agility; limber; flexible.

surfer's knobs

Tumorlike growths of connective tissue just below the knees, on the tops of the feet, and often on the toes; common among surfers who paddle in a kneeling position; also called surfer's knee.

sweat

To excrete perspiration through the pores in the skin; perspire. Sweat is important during exercise because its evaporation helps to cool the skin and keep the body temperature down.

sweatband

A strip of absorbent cloth, usually cotton, about 1½ inches wide that is placed around the head or wrists to keep sweat from dripping into the eyes or on hands during exercise.

sweat clothes

A combination of sweat shirt and sweat pants; often matched in color and style (see *sweat shirt* and *sweat pants*).

sweat gland

Any of the numerous small, tubular glands in man that are found nearly everywhere in the skin and secrete perspiration externally through the pores.

sweat pants

A warm pair of pants, most often cotton but sometimes rubber or plastic, designed for warming up for exercise and for wear during outdoor exercise in cold weather; may have a drawstring or elastic waist with elastic cuffs.

sweat shirt

A warm shirt, most often cotton, but sometimes rubber or plastic, designed for warming up for exercise and for wear during outdoor exercise in cold weather; may have a hood with a drawstring.

swell

To increase in size or volume as a result of internal pressure; expand.

sympathetic nervous system

The part of the autonomic nervous system that controls alertness, heart rate, blood flow, blood pressure, and metabolism.

synapse

The point at which a nerve impulse passes from an axon of one neuron to the dendrite of another.

systole

The contraction of the heart that forces the blood through the circulatory system.

systolic amplitude

The measure of the proportionate velocity of the left ventricular contraction of the heart; a low amplitude can indicate a weak heart muscle; high amplitudes are associated with heart vigor and endurance.

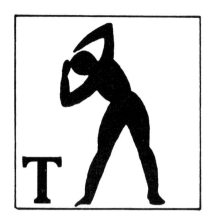

tachycardia
A heart rate exceeding 100 beats per minute; also a fluttering heart.

tactile
Perceptible to the sense of touch.

tarsus
The section of the vertebrate foot between the leg and the matatarsus, or middle foot; the seven bones making up this section.

tendonitis
Inflammation of the tendons caused by disease or overuse as with tennis elbow.

tennis
A racquet game played on a 78' x 36' court with a net that is 3' high; two or four players hit a ball with stringed racquets; points are scored if the ball lands off the playing surface, goes into the net, or bounces two times on the surface.

tennis elbow
An inflammation of the tendon in the elbow.

tensile
Capable of being stretched or extended.

tensile strength
The resistance of a material to a force tending to tear it apart.

tensiometer

Instrument used for measuring muscular strength; originally designed to measure the tension in aircraft control cables; used to measure the strength of muscles involved in orthopedic disabilities; tests measure 38 different muscles or muscle groups; originally called cable-tension tests (see *cable-tension tests*).

testosterone

A male sex hormone produced in the testes and functioning to control secondary sex characteristics; partially responsible for development of physical strength and musculature; women have only a small amount of testosterone.

the wall

A point in long-distance running at which the muscles run out of glycogen; usually occurs after about 20 miles; symptoms are extreme fatigue, heaviness in the legs, and disorientation; made popular by marathon runners; studies show that men encounter this problem more than women; also called "hitting the wall."

thiamin

A vitamin necessary for the release of energy from carbohydrates; found in pork, liver, oysters, whole grain and enriched cereals, bread, wheat germ, brewer's yeast, and green peas.

thigh

The portion of the human leg between the hip and the knee.

thrombus

A clot blocking a blood vessel or formed in a heart cavity; produced by coagulation of the blood.

thyroid gland

The two-lobed endocrine gland found in all vertebrates; located in front of and on either side of the trachea in humans and producing the hormone thyroxin, which regulates metabolism.

tibia

The inner and larger of the two bones of the lower leg from the knee to the ankle; also called shin or shinbone.

tissue

An aggregation of morphologically and functionally similar cells.

toe raise

An exercise performed in the standing position in which the heels are raised off the floor as far as possible; strengthens the calf muscles; also called the heel raise.

toe touch

An exercise performed from the standing position, with the feet close together and the knees kept straight; the exerciser bends at the waist and touches the toes with the tips of the fingers; strengthens and limbers the hamstring muscles on the backs of the legs.

torso

The trunk or upper part of the human body.

trachea

A thin-walled tube of cartilaginous and membranous tissue descending from the larynx to the bronchi and carrying the air to and from the lungs.

"Train don't strain"

A motto proposed by William Bowerman, track and field coach at the University of Oregon; refers to the fact that it is not necessary to become physically exhausted or to suffer injury to achieve a high level of fitness; Bowerman is noted for promoting jogging as a popular fitness activity among people of all ages.

trained

A person who is in good to excellent physical condition.

training

A program of exercise designed to improve skills and increase energy capacities; for an athlete, the preparation for a particular event.

training effect

The action that occurs when the body is stressed; based on the fact that the body adapts to the level of stress that is applied continually; if that stress is increased, the body again adapts and is able to handle the heavier stress; recognized by Scandinavian physiologists in the 1930s, it later became the basis for overload training (see *overload* and *training zone*).

training heart rate

The rate that provides sufficient training for the cardiovascular system; usually between 70 and 85% of maximum (220 minus age); also called the training zone (see *training zone*).

training zone

The range to which the pulse must be raised to achieve a cardiovascular training effect; exercise that positively affects the heart must raise the pulse rate to 70% to 85% of the maximum rate; the training zone is between 70 and 85%; maximum pulse rate of an exerciser; e.g., the training pulse rate of a 20-year-old would be 170 (220-20 = 200; 85% of 200 = 170); the training zone of a 20-year-old would be 140 to 170.

trampoline

A strong, tight section of canvas attached with springs to a metal frame that suspends it off the floor; the springs allow a person to jump up and down on the canvas and perform a variety of acrobatic tumbling maneuvers; also used for fitness activities such as running in place and calisthenics.

trapezius

Either of two large, flat muscles running from the back of the head to the middle of the back; supports and makes it possible to raise the head and shoulders.

trauma

A wound, especially one produced by sudden physical injury.

treadmill

An exercise device, either motor-driven or moved by the feet, designed to allow the exerciser to run or walk in place; speed and incline can usually be adjusted to increase the intensity of the exercise.

treadmill run

See *treadmill* and *treadmill test.*

treadmill test

A test of endurance and maximum oxygen consumption that is performed on a treadmill (see *maximal oxygen consumption*).

triathlete

A person who trains for and participates in a triathlon (see *triathlon*).

triathlon

An athletic competition that requires the participants to swim, bicycle, and run a specified distance consecutively with no rest between events; though variations in distance exist, the competitors in the basic triathlon must swim 2½ miles, bicycle 112 miles, and run a marathon of 26 miles, 385 yards; the event was originally designed to test the body's maximum endurance.

triceps

The large, three-headed muscle that runs along the back of the arm behind the biceps; extends the forearm.

triceps extension

An exercise performed either sitting or standing in which the barbell or dumbbell is lowered from over the head to behind the neck and then returned to the starting position; strengthens the triceps.

triglycerides

The largest lipo-protein particles with the lowest density; lipo-proteins are a combination of triglycerides, cholesterol, phospholipids and protein; often called serum triglycerides; importance to coronary heart disease has not been clearly defined; exercise can apparently lower the level of triglycerides.

tri-set

The use of three weight training exercises for the same body segment; can include different muscles; little or no rest is allowed between exercises in the set.

trunk raise

An exercise performed while lying on the side with the legs extended; the trunk is then twisted to the right or left as the exerciser slowly raises upward to a sitting position; the trunk is lowered to the starting position and the exercise is repeated to the opposite side; strengthens the back and abdominal muscles.

Tuttle Pulse Ratio Test

The pulse rate recovery from stepping up and down on a 13-inch bench for one minute at a rate of 20 steps per minute for boys and 15 steps for girls.

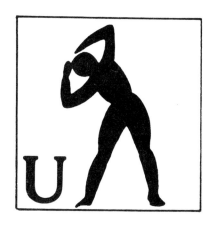

ulcer

A break in the mucous membrane, often discharging pus on the skin or an internal mucous surface of the body, resulting in the localized destruction of the tissue; often refers to stomach ulcer.

ulna

The bone extending from the elbow to the wrist on the side opposite to the thumb.

ultramarathon

Races over distances that are longer than the marathon distance of 26.2 miles; races are usually in the 40-to-80-mile range, but there are races of 100 to 500 miles and six-day races that can cover 400 to 500 miles.

underdeveloped

Not adequately or normally developed; immature, deficient; untrained.

underhand grip

The palms-out method of holding a barbell, dumbbell, or chinning bar.

underload

To work a muscle or muscle group at a load that is normally encountered in everyday life; will not produce muscular development or any physical improvement.

uneven parallel bars
Two bars of uneven height designed for use in gymnastic exercises.

unfit
A physical condition that is characterized by lack of energy, shortness of breath after moderate exercise, fatigue, and overweight; the opposite of fit.

Universal Gym
The trademark name of an exercise machine with four to sixteen exercise stations that allow the exerciser to perform a variety of weight-lifting exercises, sit-ups, dips, and other movements; suitable for use in the home.

upright row
An exercise performed by raising a barbell from the arms-extended position along the front of the body to the chin; the weight is then lowered to the starting position; hands are close together; strengthens the trapezius and deltoid muscles.

urea
A white, crystalline substance found in urine, constituting the chief nitrogenous waste product of metabolism..

U.S. Recommended Dietary Allowances
A publication of the National Research Council of the National Academy of Sciences; contains documentation for their nutritional recommendations; first published in 1943 and regularly updated (see *Recommended Dietary Allowances*).

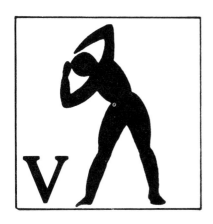

varicose

Blood or lymph vessels that are abnormally dilated, knotted, and tortuous; often visible on the legs as spidery, blue veins; can be surgically removed.

vascular

Characterized by or containing vessels for the transmission or circulation of fluids such as blood and lymph.

vascular tree

The arterial system of blood vessels and capillaries.

vasoconstriction

The constriction of a blood vessel.

vasoconstrictor

An agent, as a nerve or a drug, that causes vasoconstriction.

vasodilation

Dilation of a blood vessel.

vasodilator

An agent, as a nerve or drug, that causes vasodilation.

vasomotor

Causing or regulating vasoconstriction or vasodilation.

vaulting horse

A piece of equipment used in gymnastics; similar to a pommel horse, but used only for launching the body for a variety of athletic maneuvers (see *pommel horse*).

vegetarian

A person who eats only vegetables, grain, and dairy products; some vegetarians refrain from eating meat to protest the slaughter of animals, others for nutritional reasons; some vegetarians eat poultry and eggs, some eat fish, some refuse to eat animal products of any kind; there are approximately 10 million vegetarians in the U.S.

veggies

The term used for various kinds of vegetables, usually cut into small pieces, which are consumed in quantity by dieters and people concerned with their health.

Velcro

A special material that clings to itself and is used as a closure instead of buttons, strings, or zippers; often attached to sports clothes, sweat and wristbands, waistbands, and shoes.

ventilation

The movement of air into and out of the lungs; sometimes referred to as pulmonary ventilation and minute ventilation.

ventricle

A chamber of the heart from which blood is forced into the arteries.

vertebra

Any of the bones or cartilaginous segments forming the spinal column.

vertical jump

A strength test used in the estimate of fitness; performed by crouching into a squat position and leaping straight up to touch a spot on the wall; the higher the leap the greater the strength of the legs.

vibrator

An electrically operated device used for massage.

vital capacity
Maximal volume of air forcefully expired after a maximal inhalation.

vitamin
Any of various relatively complex organic substances occurring naturally in plant and animal tissue and essential in small amounts for the control of metabolic processes (see specific vitamins).

Vitamin A
A vitamin necessary for formation and maintenance of skin, mucous membranes, bone growth, vision, reproduction, and teeth; sources are liver, eggs, cheese, butter, milk, and vegetables (yellow, orange, and dark green); if deficient, can result in hardening and roughening of the skin, night blindness, and degeneration of mucous membranes.

Vitamin B-Complex
A group of vitamins originally thought to be a single substance, generally regarded as including thiamine, riboflavin, niacin, pantothenic acid, biotin, pyridoxine, folic acid, inositol, and Vitamin B-12 and occurs chiefly in yeast, liver, eggs, and some vegetables; a deficiency can cause problems in the nervous system or beriberi which affects the nervous system and the heart.

Vitamin B-12
Essential for the building of genetic material, formation of red blood cells, and functioning of the nervous system; found in liver, kidneys, meat, fish, eggs, milk, and oysters; a deficiency can result in anemia—a deficiency in red blood cells.

Vitamin C
For the maintenance of bones, teeth, blood vessels, and the formation of collagen, which supports body structure; found in fruits and leafy vegetables; also called ascorbic acid; a deficiency can cause scurvy—sponginess of the gums and loosening of the teeth.

Vitamin D
Any of several chemically similar activated sterols, especially

Vitamin D-2 or Vitamin D-3, produced in general by ultraviolet irradiation of sterols; obtained from milk, fish, liver, and eggs; required for normal bone growth and used to treat rickets in children and osteomalacia in adults.

Vitamin E

Any of several chemically related viscous oils; found in vegetable oils, margarine, whole grain cereal, bread, wheat germ, liver, dried beans, and green leafy vegetables; used to treat sterility and various abnormalities of the muscles, red blood cells, liver, and brain.

Vitamin G

See *riboflavin*.

Vitamin H

See *biotin*.

Vitamin K

Any of several natural and synthetic substances essential for the promotion of blood clotting and the prevention of hemorrhage; occurring naturally in leafy green vegetables, tomatoes, milk, and vegetable oils.

Vitamin P

A crystalline fraction of citrus juices used to treat certain conditions involving hemorrhage into the skin.

voluntary muscle

Muscle normally controlled by individual volition.

VO$_2$max

See *maximum oxygen uptake*.

V-sit

An exercise performed from the sitting position with the knees bent; the legs are slowly extended until they form a V with the trunk; strengthens the abdominal and thigh muscles and affects all muscle groups.

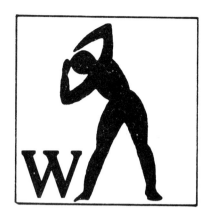

waist

The part of the human trunk between the bottom of the rib cage and the pelvis.

waist circle

An exercise performed from a standing position; circle the trunk to the left, around to the back and then to the right, completing a full circle; repeat to the right; a good stretching exercise.

Walkman

The Sony trademark name of a radio and/or tape player with earphones that is compact and light enough to be worn or carried during exercise; any of a number of other companies' adaptations of the Sony Walkman.

wall, the

See *the wall.*

warm-down

An exercise procedure (also called cool-down) performed immediately after training sessions or competitions for purposes of quickly removing any accumulated lactic acid from the muscles and blood; prevents muscle tightening and soreness; similar to warm-up routine; 5 to 15 minutes of stretching are adequate (see *warm-up*).

warm-up

A series of exercises, usually stretching movements, that gradually warm the muscles and prepare them for strenuous physical activity; used for injury prevention, joint and muscle stimulation, and psychological preparation for exercise; physiologists recommend 5 to 15 minutes of warm-ups (see *warm-downs*).

water stop

A place along a race course where water is available for runners; in organized races, stops are usually placed every 2 miles.

weight control

The process of maintaining ideal weight (see *ideal weight*).

weight-lifter's belt

A wide leather belt used for support during heavy weight lifting; fastens tightly at the waist; said to help support the back.

weight table

A list of desirable weights arranged according to height and size of body frame; developed by the insurance industry (see *ideal weight*).

weight training

The use of resistance exercises to increase the strength or endurance of the muscles; equipment for weight training can include barbells, dumbbells, or specialized exercise machines; has been found to be valuable for all sports.

Wells and Dillon Sit-and-Reach Test

A test that measures flexibility; performed while sitting on the floor; arms are stretched forward toward a mark on the floor; distance measured from the crotch to the fingertips indicates flexibility.

whirlpool bath

A type of tub in which water is rapidly moving in a circular direction; used by athletes and others for soothing the muscles following exercise or for general relaxation; found in team training facilities, health clubs, and spas; can be installed in a home tub; hot tubs are a variation on the whirlpool.

white blood cells

One of the three solid elements of the blood that are visible under an ordinary microscope (others are platelets and red blood cells); prevent infection and repair tissue; normal count ranges from 5,000 to 9,000 per cubic millimeter (see *red blood cells*).

white muscle fibers

See *fast twitch fibers*.

Witten Submaximal Step Test

A submaximal step test of alternate stepping and resting; based on the number of stepping bouts to reach a heart rate of 168 beats per minute; similar to Harvard Step Test (see *Harvard Step Test*).

work interval

That portion of an interval training program consisting of the work effort; the activity as opposed to the rest period (see *interval training program*).

workload

The amount of intensity placed on the body during exercise; e.g., running uphill creates more of a workload for the body than running on a flat surface or downhill; application of a force through a distance; for example, moving 1 kilogram through 1 meter equals 1 kilogram-meter of work.

workout

Any type of exercise activity.

wrist

The junction between the hand and forearm; the system of bones forming this junction.

wristband

A strip of absorbent cloth, usually cotton, about 2-inches wide, which is placed around the wrist to prevent sweat from dripping from the arms onto the hands during exercise; e.g., keeps hands dry for a firmer grip on the bar during weight-lifting exercises.

wrist curl

An exercise performed with a barbell or dumbbell held in the hands with the forearms resting on the thighs; the hands are extended past the knees, palms up; the weight is then curled up toward the wrists as far as possible and returned to the starting position; strengthens the wrists and forearms; can also be done with palms down (called reverse wrist curl).

wrist roller

A handle with a rope attached and a weight suspended at the bottom of the rope; using the wrists and forearms, the weight is rolled up on the handle; strengthens the wrists and forearms.

wrist weights

Light weights wrapped around the wrist and attached by a buckle or velcro fastener; used to add resistance.

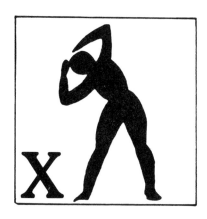

XBX Program

A progressive schedule of ten calisthenic exercises for women developed by the Royal Canadian Air Force (see *Royal Canadian Air Force Plans for Physical Fitness*).

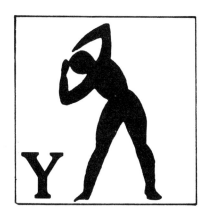

YMCA

The Young Men's Christian Association; among the first public health and fitness facilities; offers swimming, weight lifting, boxing, and gymnastics to all; the Young Women's Christian Association (YWCA) and the Young Men's and Young Women's Hebrew Association (YM-YWHA) also offer these services.

yoga

A Hindu discipline aimed at training the consciousness for a state of perfect spiritual insight and tranquility; a system of exercises practiced as a part of this discipline to promote control of the body and mind (see *asana*).

York Barbell Company

One of the first barbell manufacturing companies; located in York, PA.; founded by Bob Hoffman; sponsors weight lifters and weight-lifting teams who train at a facility on the company grounds; York Barbell Club was prominent in the world of international weight lifting in the 1940s and 1950s; a body-building museum is sponsored by the company.

"You're looking good"

A term of encouragement often shouted to runners by spectators at various stages of a long-distance race.

DIAGRAMS

MUSCULAR SYSTEM

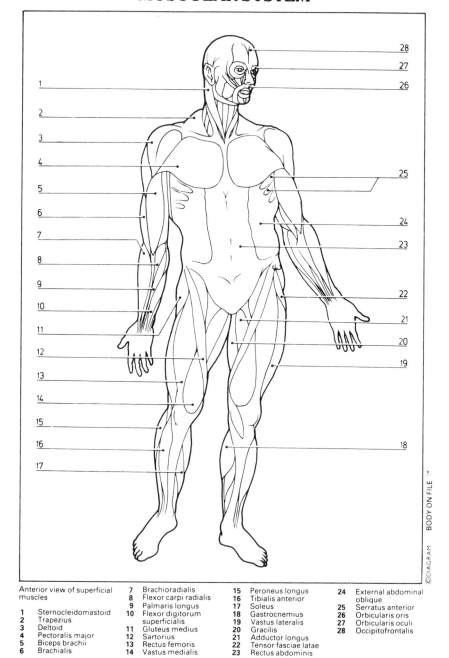

Anterior view of superficial muscles

1 Sternocleidomastoid
2 Trapezius
3 Deltoid
4 Pectoralis major
5 Biceps brachii
6 Brachialis
7 Brachioradialis
8 Flexor carpi radialis
9 Palmaris longus
10 Flexor digitorum superficialis
11 Gluteus medius
12 Sartorius
13 Rectus femoris
14 Vastus medialis
15 Peroneus longus
16 Tibialis anterior
17 Soleus
18 Gastrocnemius
19 Vastus lateralis
20 Gracilis
21 Adductor longus
22 Tensor fasciae latae
23 Rectus abdominis
24 External abdominal oblique
25 Serratus anterior
26 Orbicularis oris
27 Orbicularis oculi
28 Occipitofrontalis

©DIAGRAM   BODY ON FILE ™

MUSCULAR SYSTEM

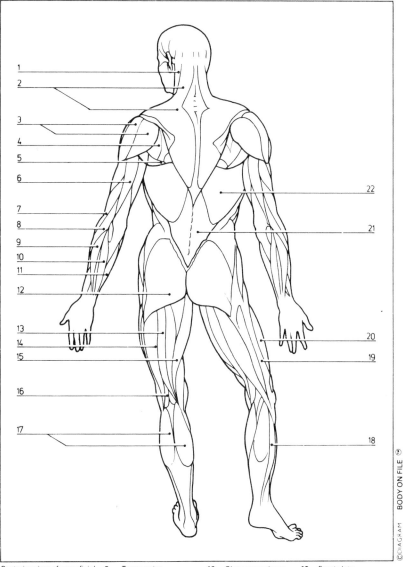

Posterior view of superficial muscles	5	Teres major	12	Gluteus maximus	19	Fascia lata
	6	Triceps brachii	13	Biceps femoris	20	Vastus lateralis
	7	Brachioradialis	14	Semitendinosus	21	Thoracolumbar fascia
1 Sternocleidomastoid	8	Extensor carpi radialis	15	Gracilis	22	Latissimus dorsi
2 Trapezius	9	Extensor digitorum	16	Semimembranosus		
3 Deltoid	10	Extensor digiti minimi	17	Gastrocnemius		
4 Infraspinatus	11	Extensor carpi ulnaris	18	Soleus		

155

CARDIOVASCULAR SYSTEM

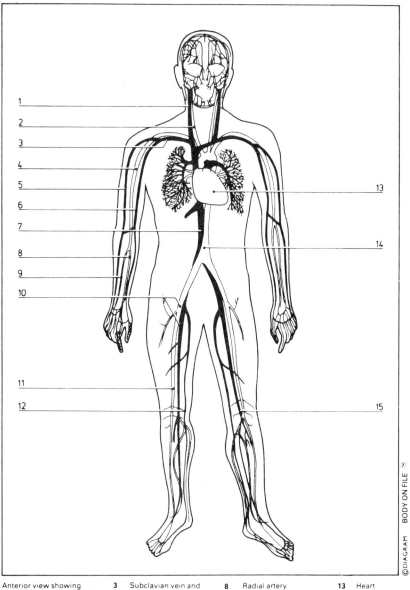

Anterior view showing major arteries (white) and veins (black)

1	Internal jugular vein
2	Common carotid artery
3	Subclavian vein and artery
4	Brachial artery
5	Cephalic vein
6	Basilic vein
7	Inferior vena cava
8	Radial artery
9	Ulnar artery
10	Common iliac artery and vein
11	Femoral artery
12	Great saphenous vein
13	Heart
14	Aorta
15	Femoral vein

©DIAGRAM   BODY ON FILE ™

RESPIRATORY SYSTEM

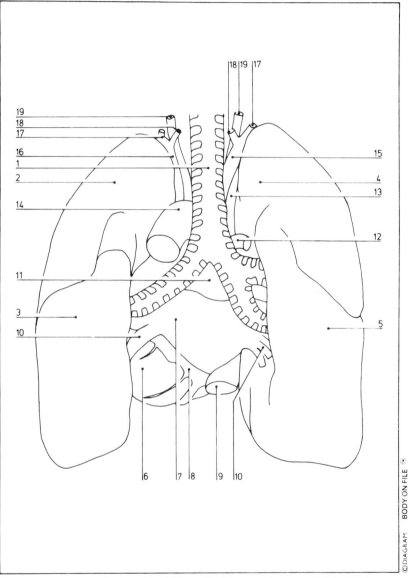

		18	19	17

19
18
17
16
1
2
14
11
3
10

15
4
13
12
5

|6 |7 |8 |9 |10

©DIAGRAM   BODY ON FILE ©

Posterior view	**5**	Lower lobe of right lung	**10**	Pulmonary veins	**16**	Left subclavian artery
1 Trachea	**6**	Left ventricle	**11**	Pulmonary artery	**17**	Thyrocervical trunks
2 Upper lobe of left lung	**7**	Left atrium	**12** ·	Azygos vein	**18**	Vertebral arteries
3 Lower lobe of left lung	**8**	Coronary sinus	**13**	Superior vena cava	**19**	Common carotid arteries
4 Upper lobe of right lung	**9**	Inferior vena cava	**14**	Aorta		
			15	Brachiocephalic trunk		

157

SKELETAL SYSTEM

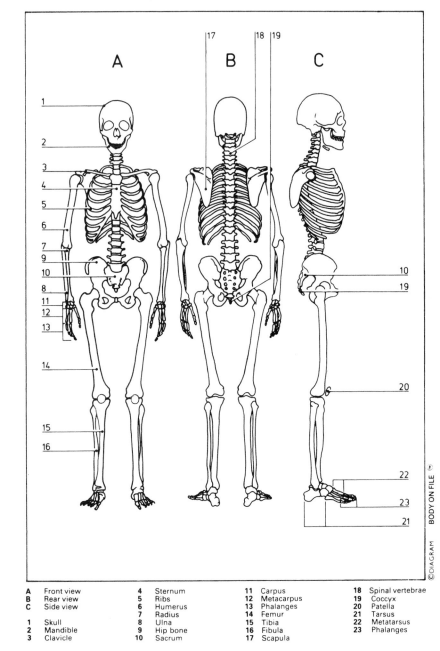

A	Front view	4	Sternum	11	Carpus	18	Spinal vertebrae
B	Rear view	5	Ribs	12	Metacarpus	19	Coccyx
C	Side view	6	Humerus	13	Phalanges	20	Patella
		7	Radius	14	Femur	21	Tarsus
1	Skull	8	Ulna	15	Tibia	22	Metatarsus
2	Mandible	9	Hip bone	16	Fibula	23	Phalanges
3	Clavicle	10	Sacrum	17	Scapula		